CONCORD
GT2290.H317
HAIRSTYLES AND H

Y0-DLX-160

3 4211 000035565

DATE DUE

DEMCO 38-297

Hairstyles and Hairdressing

Hairstyles and Hairdressing

Molly Harrison

Illustrated by Elizabeth Clarke

Dufour 1969

KLINCK MEMORIAL LIBRARY
Concordia Teachers College
River Forest, Illinois 60305

© Molly Harrison 1968
Dufour Editions, Inc.
Chester Springs
Pennsylvania 19425

Set in 12 point Monotype Bembo

Printed by Ebenezer Baylis and Son Ltd
The Trinity Press, Worcester, and London

Contents

    Read this first 7

1. Styles for men and boys in the 17th century 9
2. Styles for women and girls in the 17th century 17
3. Styles for men and boys in Georgian times 22
4. Styles for women and girls in Georgian times 28
5. Styles for men and boys 1800–1914 34
6. Styles for women and girls 1800–1914 37
7. Hairstyles since the Great War 44
8. How do we know? 48
9. Hairdressing as a career 53
10. Your own hair 62

    Finding out for yourself 67

    Index 69

Acknowledgments

The author and publishers wish to thank the following for their help in providing the photographs which illustrate this book:

Brighton Museum *page 48*; British Museum *page 51 bottom, page 57*; Ceylon Tea Centre *page 31 right*; Reverend G. Hill *page 51 top right*; National Portrait Gallery *page 49*; Oxford University Press *page 54*; Radio Times Hulton Picture Library *pages 21, 30, 31 left, 41, 43, 58, 61, 65*; Rex Features *page 47 right*; S. K. R. Photos *page 47 left*; Sotheby and Co. *page 16*; Victoria and Albert Museum *page 51 top left*; Charles Woollett and Son *page 50*.

Read this first

Your hair is one of the most important parts of you. It is what people usually notice first, and if you know that your hair looks neat and attractive you usually feel good.

Nowadays there is a hairdresser's in nearly every shopping street, and people of all kinds spend a lot of time and money on their hair. This used not to be so, as we shall see, and until recently you could not have a fashionable hairstyle, or smart clothes either, unless you were rich.

We all get ideas about how to dress, and how to do our hair, from looking at other people or at pictures of them. Men and women seem always to have wanted to try out new ways of arranging and cutting and decorating their hair. Probably it was an enterprising cave woman who first started it, when she decided that she looked nicer when she tied her hair back with a piece of stalk or grass, instead of having it hanging over her eyes. Since then, both men and women have arranged their hair in an astonishing variety of ways, and this book is about some of those ways.

We are going to look at hairstyles which have been worn in England during the past three hundred years. But do remember that we shall be talking about, and looking at wealthy, smart people. We know really very little about how the ordinary people looked, and anyway they were certainly too poor and too busy to have a great deal of time for fashion.

While you are reading these chapters and looking at the pictures, try to decide *how* we know what people looked like, and what their hairstyles were, so long ago. Later, we shall discuss this, but perhaps you can decide some of it for yourself beforehand too.

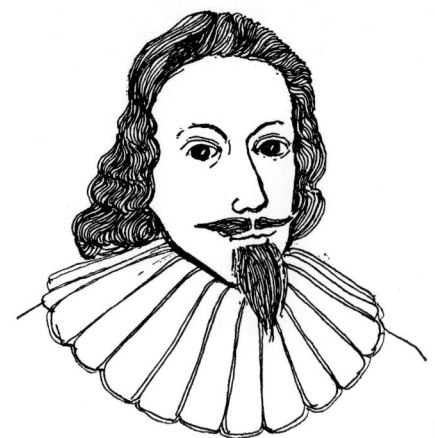

Early seventeenth century

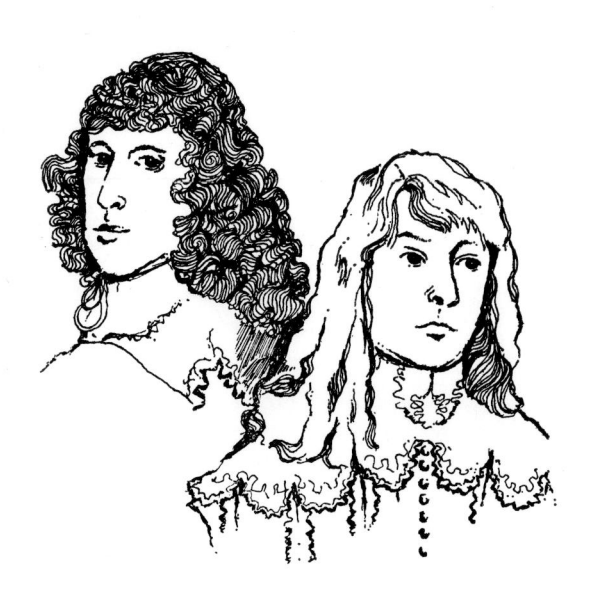

Young men in 1637

CHAPTER ONE

Styles for men and boys in the 17th century

Most boys and girls have fierce arguments with their parents about their hair. Perhaps your father or mother does not like a new style you are trying out, or a new colour; maybe they think your hair is not clean enough, or perhaps the complaint is that it is too long.

There is nothing new about any of this. Parents have probably always argued about their children's looks, and perhaps that cave woman's husband did not like it when she looked different from the other women living in the same area. At times teachers, too, have complained and have made rules about the length of hair that their pupils could wear in school.

It was not only parents and teachers who decided how young people should wear their hair in the seventeenth century. In 1603, the year in which Queen Elizabeth I died, the magistrates in Newcastle gave instructions that apprentices in the town must not 'weare their hayre long, nor locks at the ears like ruffians'. If they disobeyed, they were sent to prison; but in a few months the law was dropped, because there were so many long-haired apprentices that the court was too busy to deal with them!

And in 1636 boys going to Harvard College, in the new American Colony, were instructed 'nor shall it be permitted to wear long hair, locks, curlings, partings or powdering of the hair'.

Nowadays, one of the criticisms which boys and young men sometimes have to put up with is that they wear their hair in a girlish way. This is often said in an unkind way, as if it were rather disreputable for a man to wear a style that we think of as being feminine. But there is certainly nothing wrong and nothing new in this, and people who criticize must have

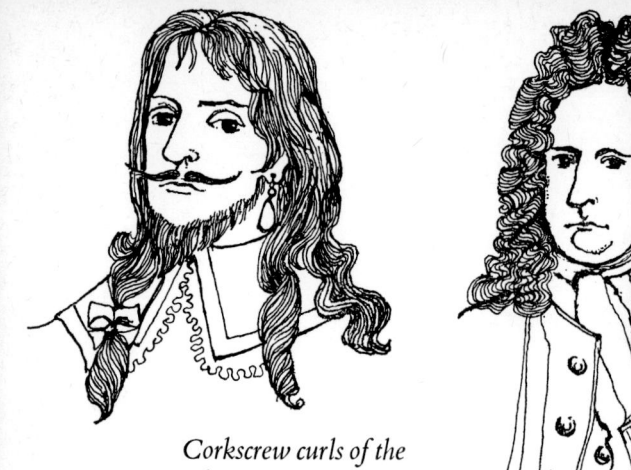

Corkscrew curls of the 1630s

Late seventeenth century styles

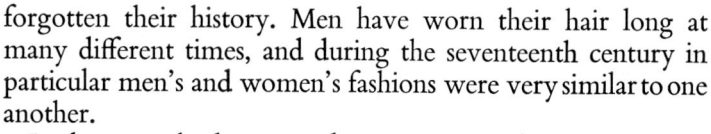

forgotten their history. Men have worn their hair long at many different times, and during the seventeenth century in particular men's and women's fashions were very similar to one another.

In the 1630s both men and women wore their hair in long corkscrew curls hanging down the back and over the shoulders. In the 1670s men wore theirs flatter on top with the curls frizzed out at the side of the head, just as women did. And in the 1690s it was very fashionable for both men and women to have a centre parting and to pile their hair very high on top, in two peaks.

The seventeenth century in England was a time when people's opinions differed very strongly on a number of matters. They argued and fought about religion, about politics and about what were the right ways of behaving. Human beings have always argued about such things, but seventeenth-century English men and women felt so strongly that they fought the Civil War about them, and there were many fierce battles in which cousins killed one another and friend killed friend. Disagreements even went so far that the King, Charles I, was beheaded, and for everyone it was a time of very bitter feelings.

To show which side you were on at that time you wore a kind of uniform. Not a compulsory one, in the way that soldiers, policemen and nurses do nowadays, but you wore the *style* of clothes that showed your views. Men's and women's

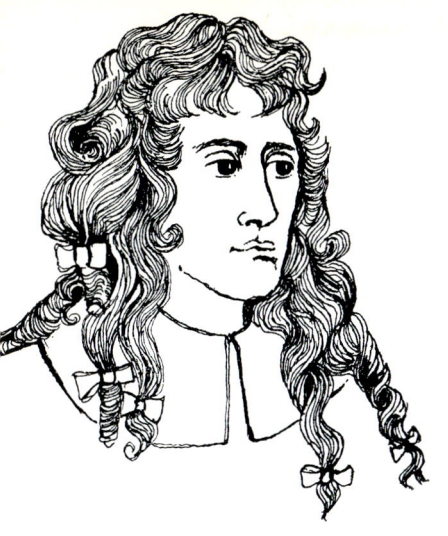

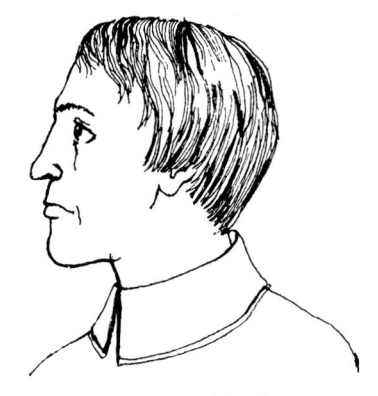

Cavalier   *Roundhead*

hairstyles also showed their views, and boys and girls wore their hair in a way which fitted in with their fathers' and mothers' opinion. If your father was on the side of the King, he was a Royalist, or Cavalier and wore elegant clothes and had his hair in long curls. If he was on the side of the Parliament and against the King, he was a Puritan and wore plainer clothes, without lace or frills, and his hair was cut short, cropped close to the head, and he was called a Roundhead—you can see why.

Not everybody showed their views as definitely as this, but it was quite normal to do so. It would seem very strange to us nowadays if Conservatives did their hair differently from Liberals or members of the Labour Party. But the differences between the political parties nowadays are not nearly as strong, nor as bitter, as the differences between Cavaliers and Roundheads were in the seventeenth century.

Puritans were mostly clean shaven, but many Cavaliers wore pointed beards and moustaches, brushed upwards into waxed points. They wore their curls of hair tied with ribbons and a fashion for wearing a 'lovelock' over one shoulder, with a pearl earring on the other ear, was introduced into England by King Charles I. The earring was attached either by a thin piece of string, or by a hook made of gold wire.

Some daring young men, we might call them 'hippies' now, began to powder their hair with fine flour during the 1640s, but the idea was soon dropped because the flour made marks on the jackets made from satin or velvet which they wore.

There was a fashion for wearing wigs and pieces of false hair from the 1660s. This fashion had started earlier in the French Court and was brought to England by King Charles II who had spent many years in exile in France after his father's execution. The word 'wig' came from the French word *perruque*, which was wrongly pronounced 'perewyke' by English people, and then gradually became 'periwig' and then 'wig' for short.

Charles II came back to England wearing, over his shaven head, a long and very splendid full-bottomed black wig, which was a mass of tumbling ringlets of different lengths. Quickly the fashion spread in England and after a time wigs were made of horsehair, which kept its curl better than human hair.

Because wigs were so hot you had to wear a small cap of linen next to your head, and you took your wig off as soon as you could when you got home, because it was pretty uncomfortable. Indoors, you wore a turban and at night a small cap of silk to protect your cropped head from draughts, and put your wig on a wooden stand.

Wigs cost a lot of money and a well-dressed gentleman would expect to have a number of them. In 1672, the account books of the Duke of Bedford show that four wigs were bought for him that year, costing twenty pounds, eighteen pounds, ten pounds and six pounds. The one costing ten pounds was described as a 'periwig for riding'. One old wig was sent by the Duke's Keeper of the Privy Purse to be cleaned

A Wig of the type worn by Charles II

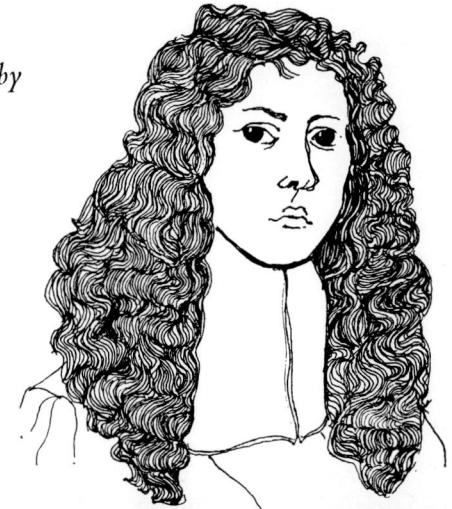

and mended, and the bill for this was ten shillings. As time went on the Duke had fewer new periwigs and had his old ones mended more often, either because he was getting older and did not worry so much about keeping up appearances, or because wigs were not so fashionable.

Towards the end of the seventeenth century white wigs came into fashion and men began to dust them with a powder made of wheat flour or sifted starch, mixed with plaster of Paris. They often added scent to their hair powder and patted pomade, a kind of paste, on to the wig to help the powder stick on. Of course, all this added to the expense and if you were not rich you were unlikely to have a wig at all, unless you were lucky enough to get hold of one that somebody had thrown out.

1720. One gentleman is wearing his wig, the others have taken theirs off. Can you see them?

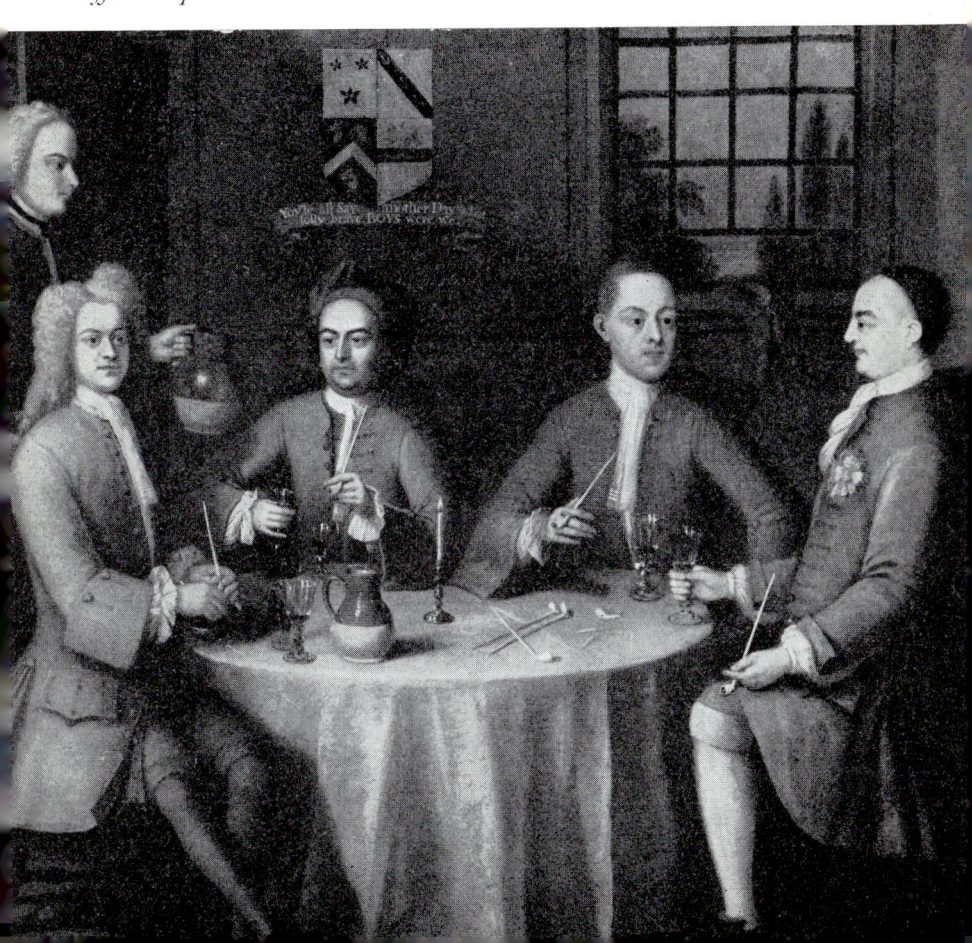

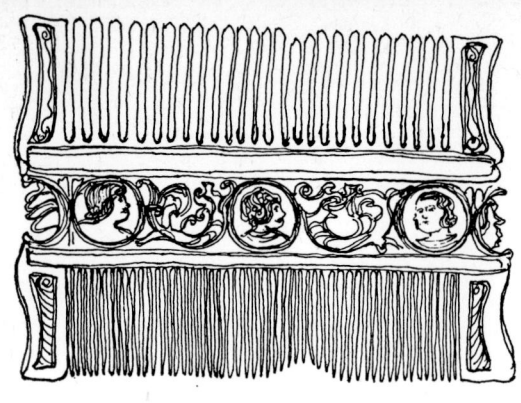

A sixteenth century ivory comb

Wealthy people, living in grand houses, had a special little room called a 'powdering room' in which they kept their wigs and a kind of thin coat which they put on over their clothes while the wig was being 'dressed'. We still speak of 'dressing' hair, and of going to the 'hairdresser's', even if all we have done there is cutting. And we still speak of our 'dressing' gown, although we do not dress ourselves in it.

The curls in a wig were tightened by rolling tufts of hair over small sausage-shaped tubes of clay, which had been heated. They looked very much like the rollers that women and girls have been using during the past few years, but were much heavier.

Elegant gentlemen carried large combs of ivory, silver or tortoiseshell, in handsome cases, in the pockets of their coats. It was considered quite polite to comb your hair or your wig in public, and Samuel Pepys was certainly not the only gentleman in the seventeenth century who employed his wife's maid to brush his hair for him each evening. On 31st May, 1662 he wrote in his diary:

> Had Sarah to comb my hair clean, which I found so foul with powdering and other troubles, that I am resolved to try if I can keep my hair dry without powder; and I did also in a suddaine fit cut off all my beard, which I had been a great while bringing up (growing) . . . she also washed my feet in a bath of herbs, and so to bed.

Men used perfume not only because it was smart, but also to disguise the smell of tobacco pipe smoking, which was a new and very fashionable thing to do. The smell of stale tobacco on a person's clothes or in their breath was unpleasant then, as it still is now. It seems surprising that seventeenth-century people noticed the smell of tobacco, but not the smell of dirty bodies. They washed themselves very rarely and it was quite normal to see lice and fleas on a person's clothes or face and neck.

When large, heavy wigs were fashionable men tended to carry their hats rather than to wear them, so as not to disarrange the curls. This may have been the beginning of the custom of taking off your hat indoors. There are paintings which show us courtiers wearing their hats at table in the seventeenth century, but the custom had evidently disappeared by the eighteenth century.

A boy in 1650

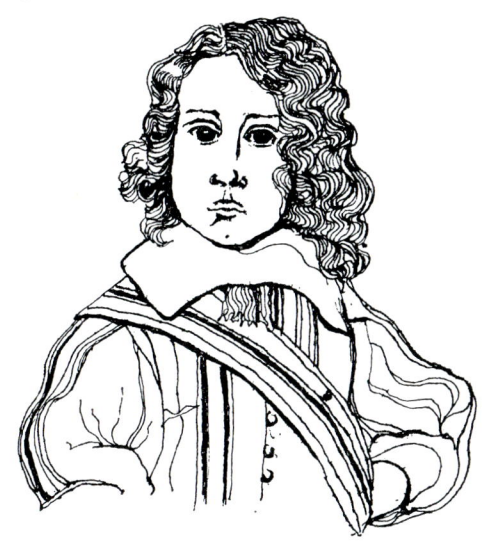

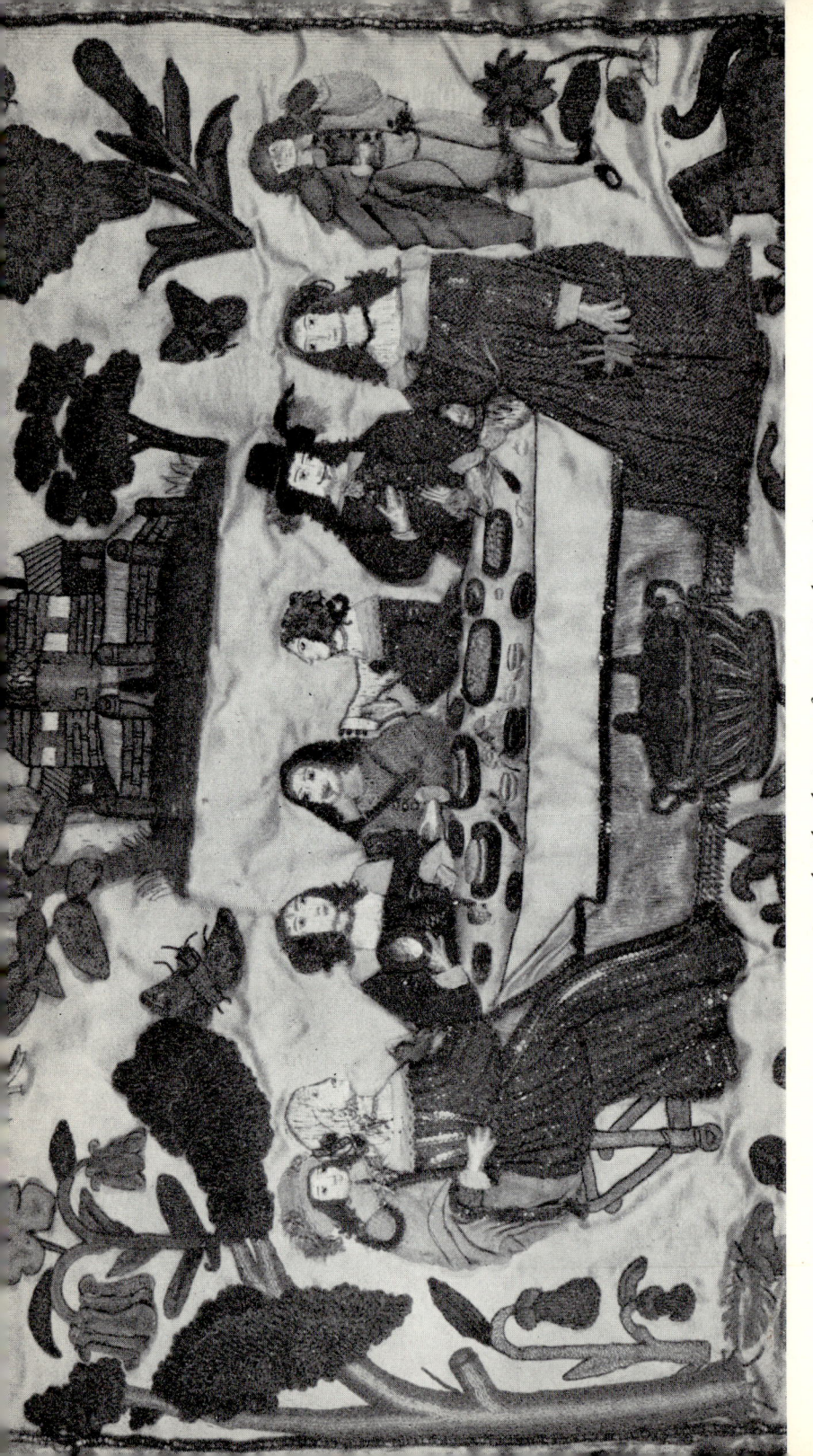

An embroidered picture of a party in about 1640

CHAPTER TWO

Styles for women and girls in the 17th century

During the early part of the seventeenth century a smart lady wore her hair pulled back and arranged over a wire frame. In the front she wore a jewelled brooch fixed to a large hairpin, and on top a halo-shaped head-dress made of gauze or net, with a black velvet edging. If her hair was thin she wore a false piece or even a 'head', which was really a wig, but the name 'wig' was not yet known in England.

This rather stiff way of doing your hair went well with the very stiff dresses of the time, but fashion soon became more relaxed and graceful and in the 1630s—the time of King Charles I—hair was dressed much lower, with a fringe and with a lot of ringlets. Some ladies wore their curls over their cheeks; others crimped them at the sides so they stuck out in a kind of bush, and this was called the 'sheep style' for obvious reasons! It was smart, too, to wear a curl over one shoulder, which was called a love-lock. Kiss-curls were tiny ringlets at the back of the neck.

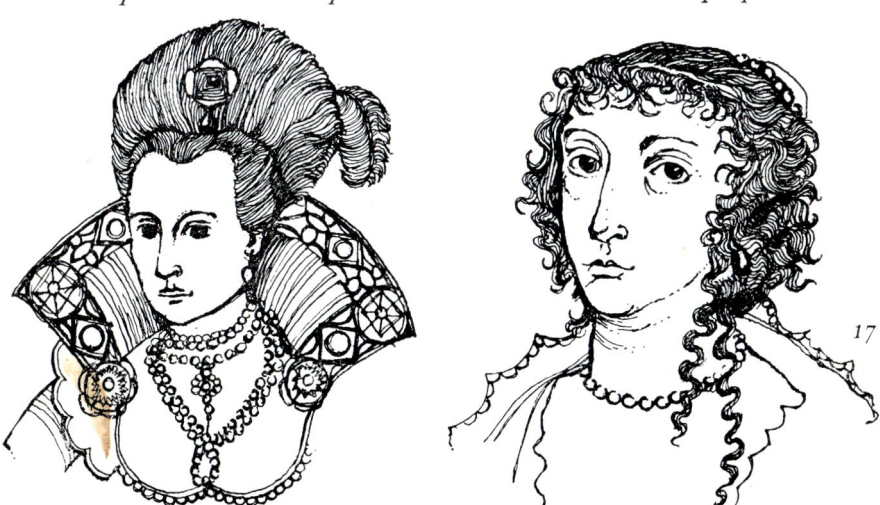

Early seventeenth century

'Sheep style'

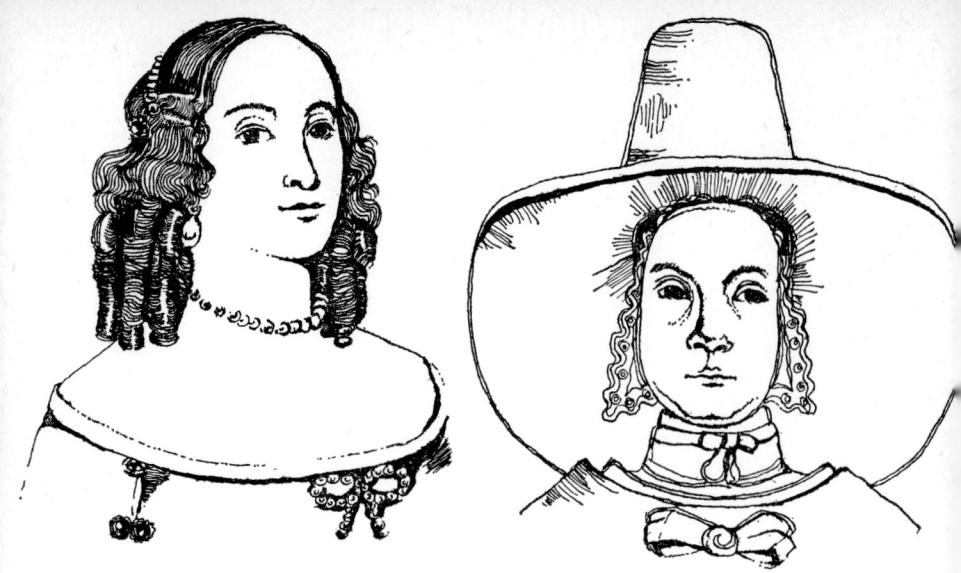

Royalist lady   *Puritan lady*

Gradually the ringlets were worn longer; strings of pearls were wound in the hair; or a bunch of flowers or a drooping feather were fixed at the side of the head.

Puritan ladies thought that too much attention should not be paid to a person's appearance. Many of them wore middle partings, brushed their hair back severely and wore a white cap under a tall, dark felt hat. Not all Puritan ladies were so strict, however, and Oliver Cromwell's own daughter wore small ringlets and bows in her hair. It depended upon your views, and your husband's views, how strict you were in your style of dress.

Royalist ladies whose husbands were active in the King's cause dressed very extravagantly, and wore their hair in long curls and ringlets covering their shoulders. Ribbon bows were very popular and jewels were twisted in the curls and in the bun at the back. If your hair was not thick enough or long enough to wear in curls you could wear false curls tied to your head with ribbons, or fixed with small combs.

Two very exaggerated styles were fashionable for a time in the 1670s: the 'hurluberlu', with the sides cut at uneven lengths, puffed out over a wire frame and crimped into two long curls, one over each shoulder; and the 'cabbage head', with large bunches of little curls dressed on either side of the forehead.

Exaggerated fashions, of any kind, are always followed by a

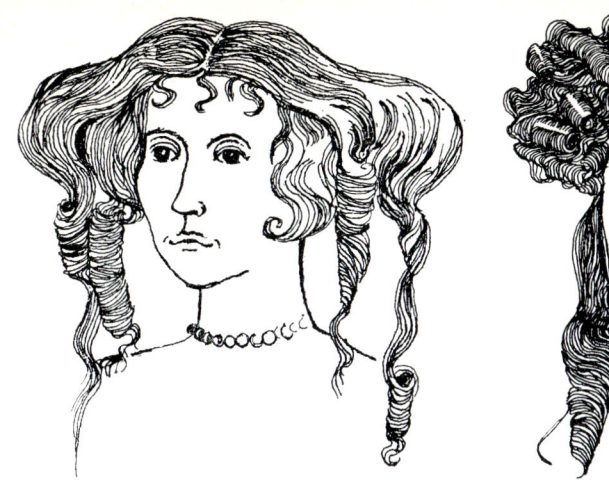

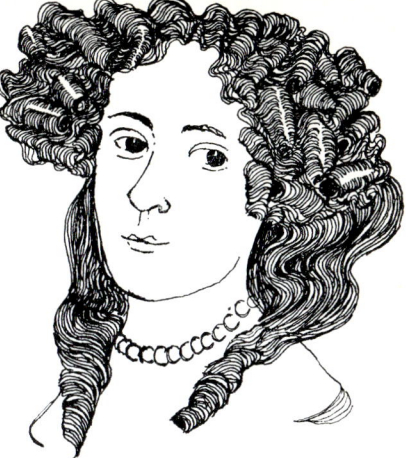

'Hurluberlu'   *'Cabbage head'*

complete change, and after some time the 'hurluberlu' and the 'cabbage head' both went out and you thought it more attractive to make your head look as narrow as possible, and to heap curls on top.

This complete change of fashion is said to have happened when, in 1675, the Duchesse de Fontanges, a favourite of King Louis XIV of France, was out hunting with the King and his courtiers. During the hunt her hat blew off in the wind and her hair tumbled down over her shoulders. She quickly tied up her curls with a lace ribbon, with the bow in front, and rode on. The King was so pleased with her appearance that she decided to do her hair that way always, and the 'ribbon of convenience' became the rage.

This high curled style of hair, with ribbon loops in front was called the 'fontanges' style after the pretty Duchess, and the bonnet of the same shape which came out a few years later was called 'the fontange' or tower cap. Sometimes a wire

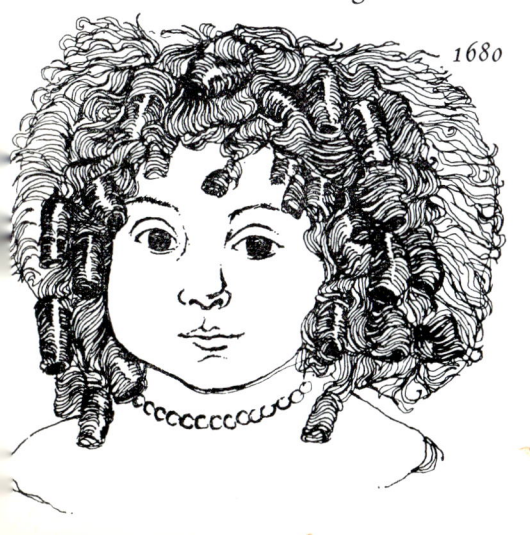

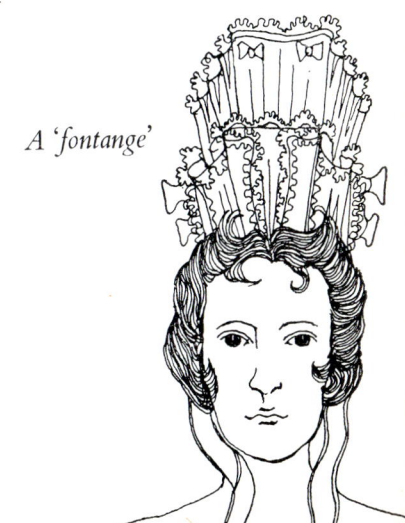

1680   *A 'fontange'*

frame was worn under curls, and the fontage cap was built up of pleated bands of lace with jewels on top. The most elaborate fontanges took a long time to make and cost up to £2,000—and money was worth *much more* three hundred years ago than it is now.

It was very difficult to walk through a doorway in an elegant way if you wore a fontange, and it was quite impossible to sit in a Sedan chair unless you had the roof raised, and then your head stuck out of the top!

One of the things that it is difficult for us to remember about the men and women who wore the elegant, charming garments which we admire in portraits, is that they must have *smelt* horrible. Most people nowadays grow up knowing that germs thrive in dirt and dust and that they cause disease. Nobody knew anything about that until a famous Frenchman, Louis Pasteur and a famous Englishman, Lord Lister, discovered the existence of germs, or bacteria, in the nineteenth century and began to think of ways of *preventing* people from getting ill, rather than waiting until they were ill and then treating them. But these two famous men lived two hundred years after the elegant, smelly ladies and gentlemen of King Charles II's court strutted about the dirty streets of London, or were driven about in their uncomfortable coaches, with hard seats and no springs.

These fashionable ladies and gentlemen used perfume to disguise the fact that they only washed themselves very rarely, and they used make-up to disguise the marks left on their faces by smallpox—a dreadful disease which killed most of those who caught it, and 'pock marked' those who survived it. The small black velvet patches which they stuck on their faces not only covered pock marks, but were also a way of drawing attention to their best features. The patches were usually round spots, but sometimes they were cut in the shapes of stars, moons, or animals. If your family were interested in politics, you wore your patches on the left or the right side of your face, according to your views!

Women made up heavily, using rouge, white chalk, white lead and paint. 'Plumpers' were pads of soft wax which were put inside the mouth to fill out the cheeks and make you look younger. If you had very thin eyebrows you would stick on false ones usually made up from mouse skin!

Up to the seventeenth century a lady had always left the care of her hair to her maid. There were no ladies' hairdressers, and men's hair was cut and looked after by barbers, who performed minor operations as well as shaving and cutting the hair of their clients.

Hair was combed rather than brushed. Wealthy ladies used combs made of ivory or tortoiseshell or silver, but everyone else used combs made of boxwood. Sets of combs were often given as presents and in 1645 Sir Ralph Verney bought in Paris half a dozen combs in a little comb-box for his sister. On one visit to France he was asked to buy combs in Dieppe which was, apparently, the best place to buy them.

The travelling difficulties described opposite were still a problem a century later as this drawing from 1796 shows

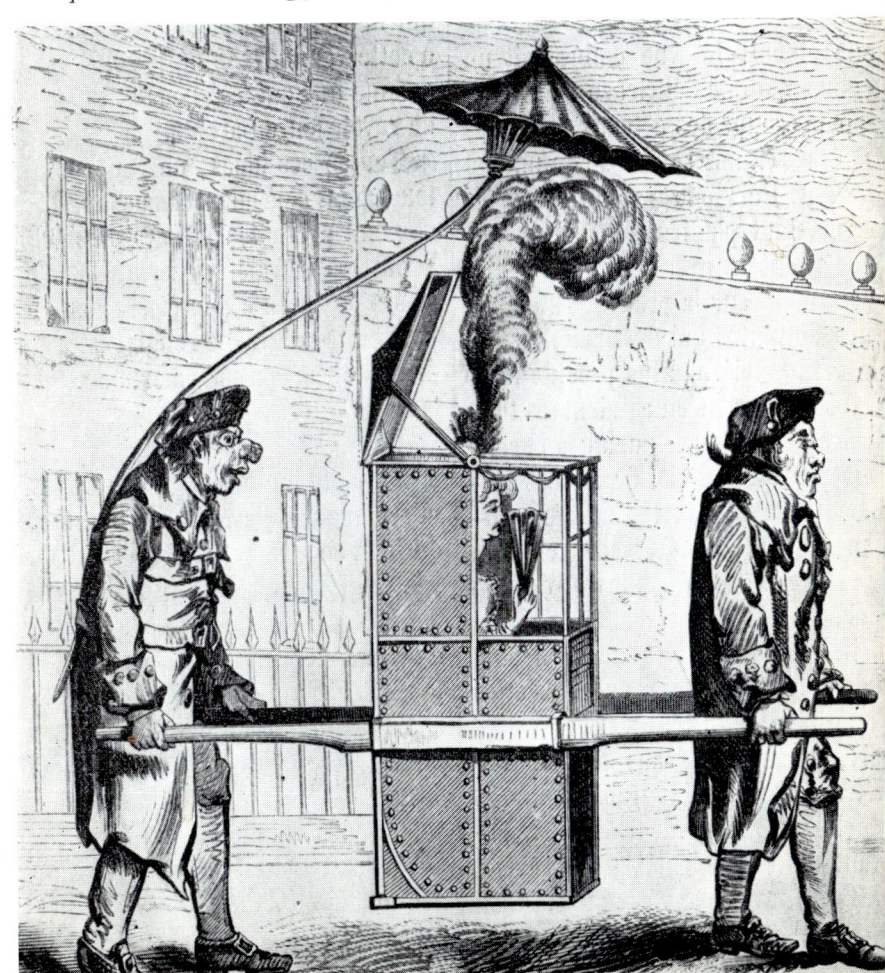

CHAPTER THREE

Styles for men and boys in Georgian times

The eighteenth century was one of the most brilliant periods in the history of costume, and during nearly the whole century a smart man wore a wig though later only for formal occasions, but no beard or moustaches. As we saw in Chapter 1, wigs were very large and very heavy by 1700, and must have been dreadfully uncomfortable to wear. Young men grew tired of the heavy wigs and began to tie them back in various ways in the summer when hunting or riding, and let them hang round their necks in winter, as this was warmer. Gradually, the large wigs went out of fashion, and only older men still wore them; if you were smart and young you tied your hair back in one of the fashionable ways:

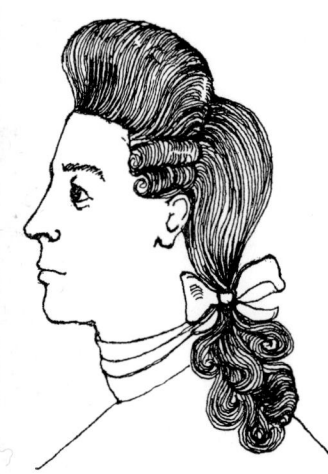

Bag wig
This was first worn by soldiers before 1700 and became general fashion in the 1730s. The front hair was brushed back and the back hair put into a black taffeta bag which was stiffened with gum. The bag was drawn up by a string and covered with a bow of the same material. In the 1740s larger bags were worn, and these protected the coat from the grease and powder of the wig.

Tie wig
The hair was drawn back and tied with a black ribbon.

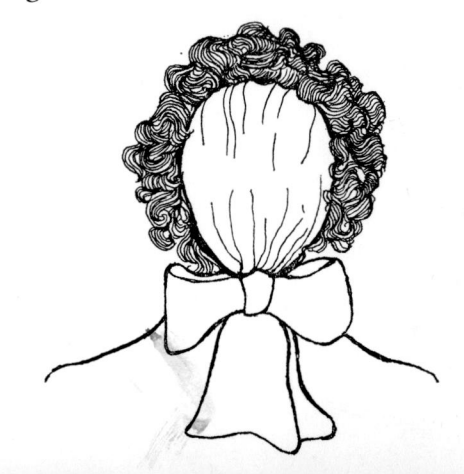

Bob wig
This was worn for everyday occasions throughout most of the eighteenth century, and was particularly popular with clergymen. A long bob covered the neck; a short bob reached to just below the ears.

Ramillies wig
This fashion was started by soldiers who had fought under the famous Duke of Marlborough against the French in the Battle of Ramillies in 1706. The back hair was plaited and fastened with a large bow at the top of the plait and a smaller one at the end.

Double-queue wig
The hair was combed away from the forehead on top, into rows of tight curls over the ears, and plaited in two plaits which hung down the back, tied with small bows in the middle. Later the plaits, or queues, were looped up and held by a comb at the back of the head.

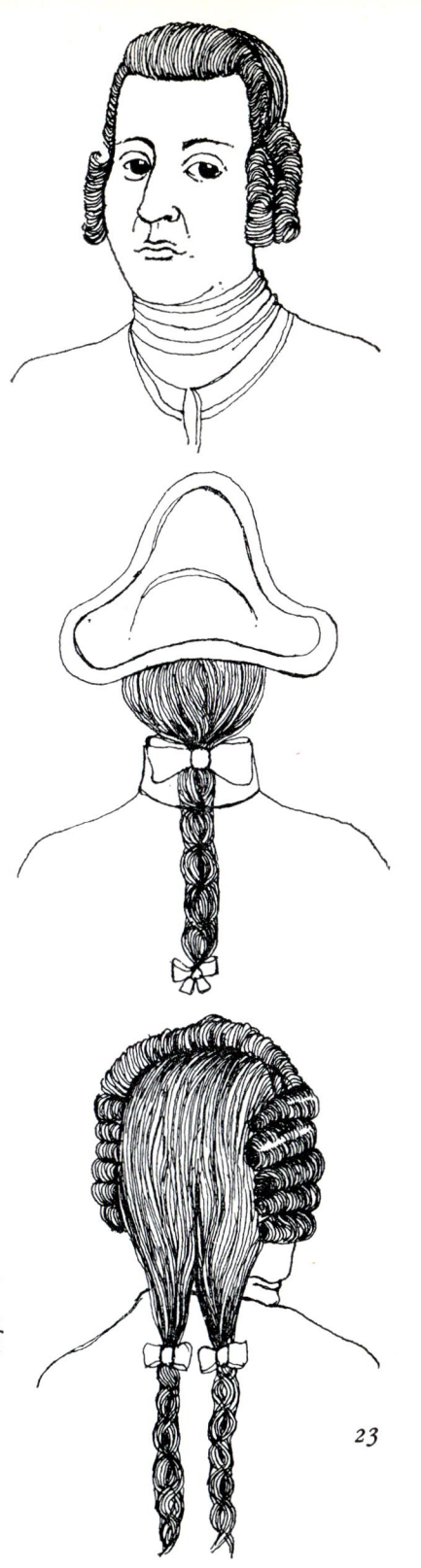

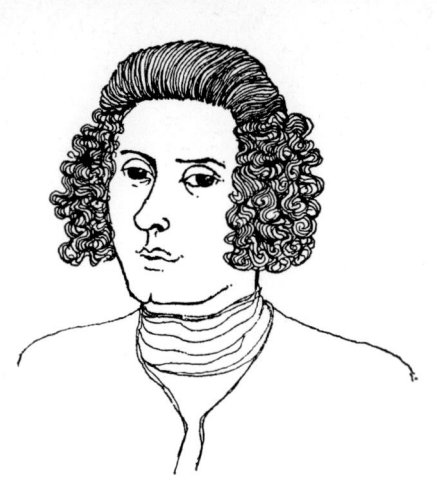

Physical wig
Worn mainly by doctors. It was very bushy, with the sides done in tight curls rolled downwards, or frizzed.

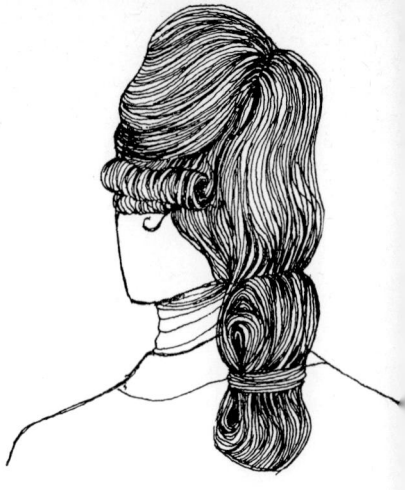

Cadogan wig
The front hair was combed back, one large roll of hair over each ear, and the long back hair looped into a large flat roll, tied at the centre.

The most exaggerated styles of hairdressing during the eighteenth century—and many were very exaggerated—were those worn by the 'macaronis'. They were a group of wealthy young men who had made what was called the 'Grand Tour' of Italy, in the 1750s, as many rich people did, visiting famous houses and collections of painting and sculpture. They came back to England in the 1760s with a passion for everything Italian and formed a club of their own, where they could meet and discuss their experiences. You can see why they called it the 'Macaroni Club'. They followed fashion in its most extreme forms, their behaviour was very eccentric and everything extreme and eccentric was named after them.

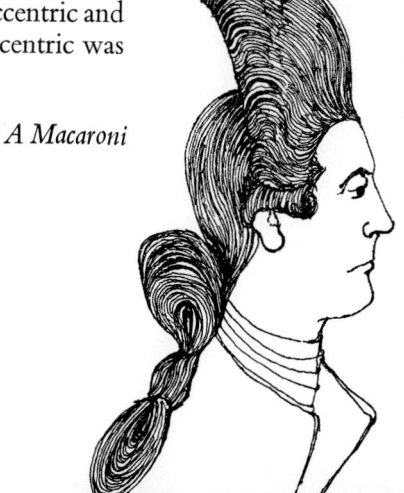

A Macaroni

White wigs were the most fashionable during much of the eighteenth century, with grey the next favourite, and all powder was made of wheat flour at first. There is an interesting story which explains how a new material for dusting wigs came to be used.

In 1715 a wealthy iron manufacturer in Germany was out riding on his horse one day when he noticed that the animal had difficulty in pulling its hooves out of the soft white earth over which they were riding. He began thinking about this and wondered whether a powder made from this earth might be useful for powdering wigs. He had some dried in his factory, tried it on his own wig, and found it was successful.

After a time this clay powder became widely used for wigs and soon a further use for it was found. One day the superintendent of a china factory at Meissen, nearby, was dusting some of the new powder on to his wig when he noticed that it was heavier than the wheat-powder he had used before. He investigated the matter and when he found out that what he was using was an earth-powder he decided to use it in making cups and bowls and so on in his factory. The result was a much more delicate clay and so now, at long last, porcelain could be made in Europe as delicate as the precious pieces that were from time to time brought by traders coming from China. It was not long before the famous English firm of Wedgwood, and others, found some of the special 'china' clay in England too and began to make white porcelain here.

The fashion for powdering the hair was at its height between 1760 and 1776 and at times pink, blue, violet and brown powders were popular, but white was always thought smartest. In France, where a great many people were very poor at that time, some fashionable people gave up using powder on their hair because of the scarcity of bread; others only used earth-powder and not wheat-powder. The famous French writer, Jean-Jacques Rousseau, once said: 'The poor are without bread because we must have powder for our hair.'

So it is not surprising that at the time of the French Revolution (1789–1795) it was no longer fashionable to wear a wig. Some older people refused to give up the custom, particularly if they were on the King's side against the Revolutionaries, and in England the Tories continued to dust their wigs, just to show that they too were against the revolution. As it had been during the English Revolution in the seventeenth century, your political views could be guessed by seeing what you wore and how you did your hair.

We know that wigs were beginning to go out of fashion as early as the 1760s, for at that time the Master Peruke Makers of London sent a petition to King George III, complaining that gentlemen were beginning to wear their natural hair, and that this made it more and more difficult to make a living from selling wigs. But the fashion was a long time in dying out, and only stopped altogether when a heavy tax was put on hair powder in 1795 and at the same time a poor wheat harvest sent up the cost of powder.

Untidily worn, natural hair became fashionable at the end of the century. In the 'hedgehog' style your hair was brushed into untidy spikes—the untidier the better. In the 'Brutus crop' you tried to have a wind-blown look.

Certain kinds of people continued to wear wigs for a long time after the eighteenth century, and some still do today. Doctors and Clergymen wore bob wigs until the early nineteenth century, and of course Judges and Barristers and Royal Coachmen still wear them on formal occasions nowadays. Look at pictures and see if you can decide when the wigs remaining today were fashionable, instead of being just a kind of uniform as they now are.

When a man decided not to wear a wig regularly any more he had, of course, to grow his own hair again. If it was not long enough to tie back in the fashionable 'queue' he wore a false one. In the French and German armies at that time, you were not allowed to wear your queue beyond a certain length, and you had to have two buttons sewn to the waist of your uniform jacket, at the back, to mark the point where the end of the queue had to be! Do you know any kind of men's jackets which still have buttons placed there?

There is one British regiment which still wears a reminder of the eighteenth century wig, as a part of their uniform. These are the Royal Welsh Fusiliers, who always wear a 'flash', or bunch of black ribbons, attached to the back of the collars of their tunics.

In the eighteenth century there were two small pieces of

furniture which were specially connected with peoples' looks. When you were not wearing your wig you kept it on a wig stand, so that it did not get crushed or untidy. When you were sitting by a fire you stood a pole screen in front of you so that the heat would not harm your skin or make you flush. Many pole screens were adjustable, so that they could be used by people of different heights.

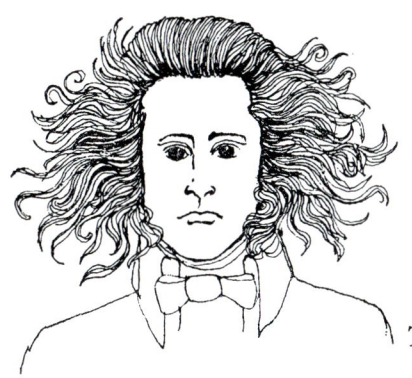

The 'hedgehog' style

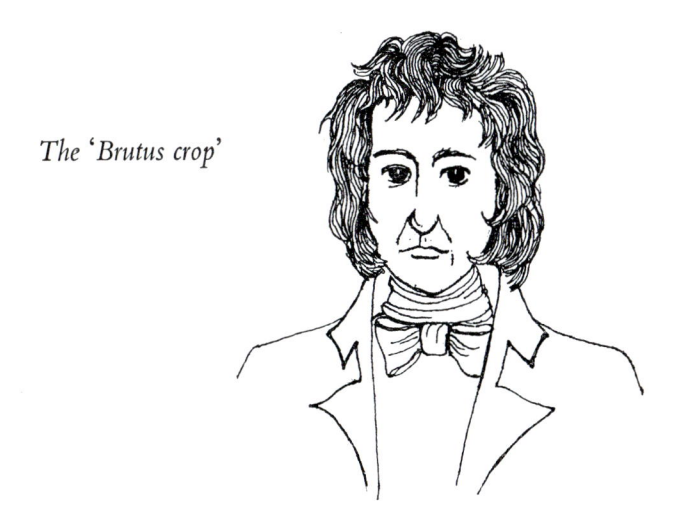

The 'Brutus crop'

CHAPTER FOUR

Styles for women and girls in Georgian times

For the first half of the eighteenth century it was smart to make your head look as small as possible. You wore your hair flat, and dressed as close to your head as you could, with the front hair drawn back off your forehead into a small topknot. You often wore a small cap made of linen or lace, and on top of that a small ornament or two, made of lace, ribbons, artificial flowers or beads.

This was called the 'Pompadour' style, after Madame de Pompadour, the very clever and beautiful mistress of King Louis XIV of France, and the leader of fashion for many years.

In the middle of the century smart ladies were keen on wearing the front of their hair in flat curls. There were French curls, English curls and Italian curls, each of different size or shape. You kept your hair flat in front and 'set' with a paste, made of flour and glue mixed together. The back hair was brushed up to the top of your head. For very dressy occasions you wore ringlets hanging down over your shoulders.

At about this time ladies began to wear wigs, just as men had

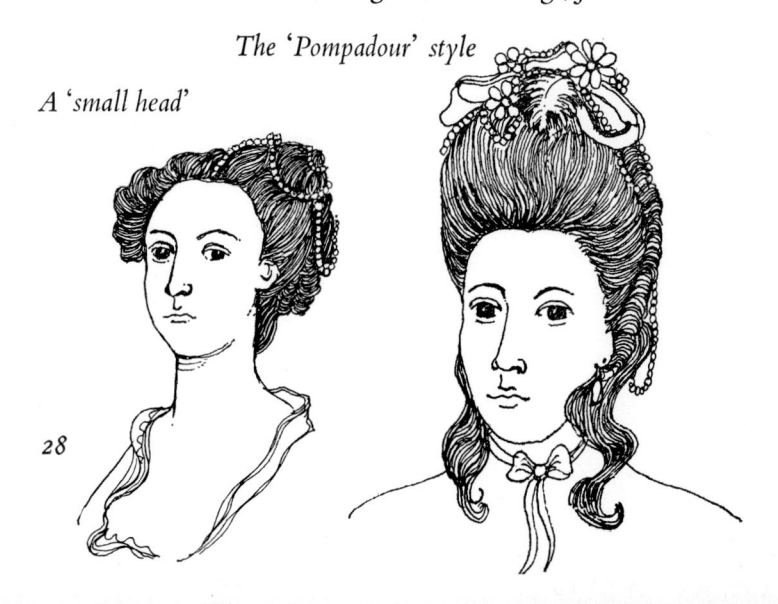

A 'small head'　　　*The 'Pompadour' style*

done for nearly a hundred years. Feminine wigs were like little caps covered with short curly hair or wool, and your own hair was dressed up over it, and ornaments fixed on top of that. It was almost impossible to do your own hair if you wore a very fashionable style; but elaborately dressed full wigs were worn by ladies who needed to be smart but had no hairdresser near, and no maid who was clever with hair.

If you were going to a ball you would need to have your hair dressed on the previous day and to sleep sitting up, so as not to disarrange it. Or you might prefer to lie down carefully, resting your neck on a little block of wood specially made to keep your head off the pillow. But in either case it seems unlikely that you would arrive for the ball looking very rested!

Powdering your hair was a complicated business, just as it was for a man. You covered your face with a kind of paper bag and the powder was blown through a tube over the hairdo, or else sprinkled on. So it is not surprising that wealthy ladies possessed a great many 'dressing' gowns and powder mantles. Grey and light brown were the favourite colours for hair powder and white was often dusted on top of another colour, to give a frosted effect. Ladies found that hair powder flattered their complexion and made their eyes look more brilliant.

An elaborate hairdo could not be taken down and rebuilt very often, so when it got dirty and smelly you had to use various kinds of perfumes and oils to disguise the smell. There are eighteenth-century advertisements describing poisons for applying to the head to kill insects. Ladies also made much use

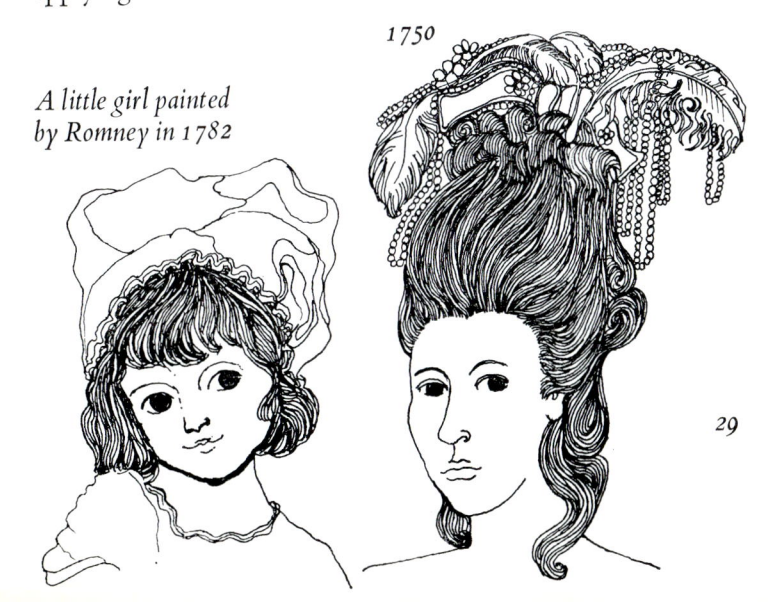

A little girl painted by Romney in 1782

1750

1785

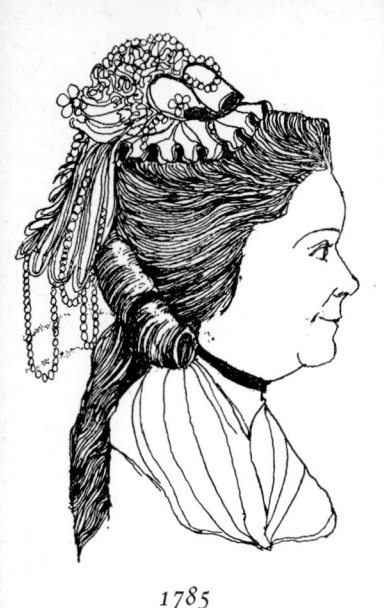

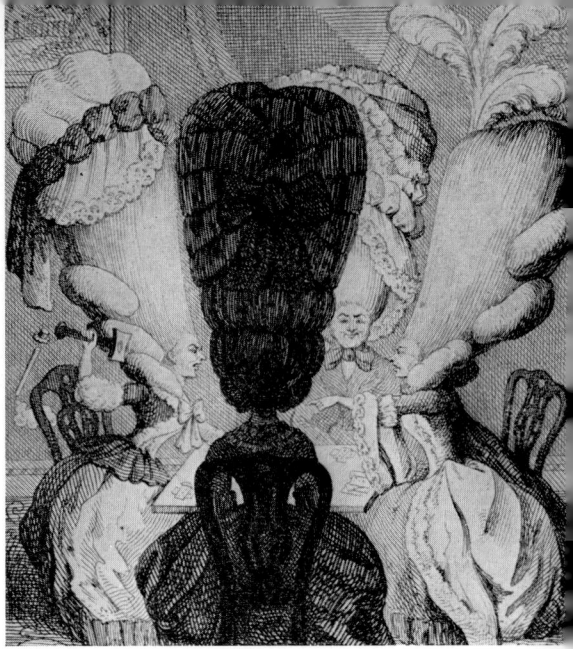

A caricature of eighteenth century hairstyles by Fairholt

of little ivory or metal 'scratchers' when their heads were irritating too much. Some scratchers had hooks on the end, others were carved in the shape of a hand, and all of them were elegant accessories for the 'dressing' table.

In the 1770s and 1780s fashionable hairstyles were so very elaborate that they became ridiculous. Your hair was built up over a cap-wig, as before, or perhaps over a horsehair cushion, a wire frame or a pad of cotton wool, to make it as high as possible. Then bits of false hair, called 'puffs' were added, and all kinds of ornaments, such as artificial flowers, jewels, ribbons, lace and feathers. A very fashionable lady would put a model ship on top, or a coach and horses, or a windmill made in blown glass. If you wanted to wear fresh flowers in your hair you hid small flat glass bottles of water among your locks!

A very thin kind of silk net called 'tulle' was a new material in the 1770s and it became very smart to wear it in strips or folds hanging down from your hair. Feathers were the rage too, especially peacock and ostrich feathers.

On several occasions ladies died from burns, when their tall head-dresses caught fire from brushing against a chandelier as they walked by. Many jokes were made about such extravagant and dangerous fashions, and in 1777 a writer composed this verse which was printed in the *London Magazine*.

Give Chloe a bushel of horse-hair and wool,
    Of paste and pomatum a pound,
Ten yards of gay ribbon to deck her sweet skull,
    And gauze to encompass it round.
Of all the bright colours the rainbow displays,
    Be those ribbons which hang on the head;
Be her flounces adapted to make the folks gaze,
    And about the whole work be they spread;
Let her flaps fly behind for a yard at the least;
    Let her curls meet just under her chin;
Let these curls be supported, to keep up the jest,
    With an hundred, instead of one pin.

Two more caricatures from contemporary engravings

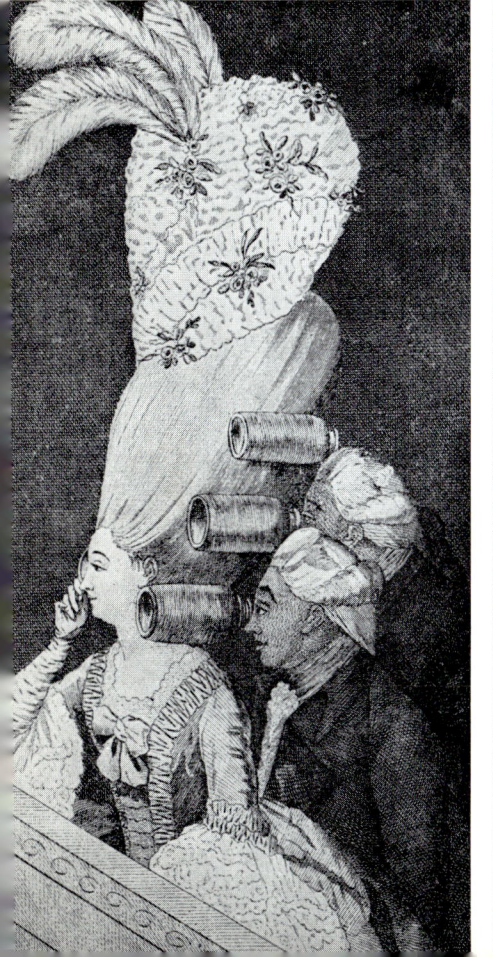

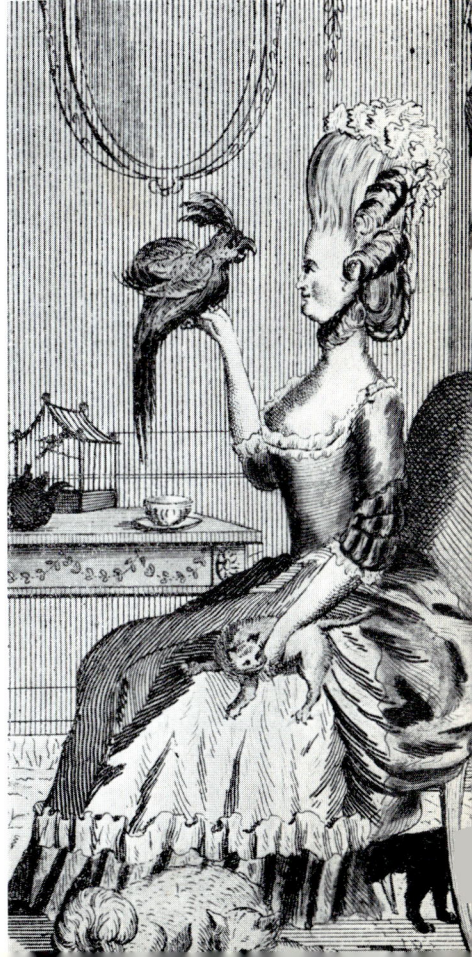

When fashions change it is usually young people who adopt the newer styles first, and this happened with hairstyles in the 1770s. The grand styles had become so elaborate and heavy that it became difficult to walk gracefully, and you had to move very slowly in case something toppled off. This did not suit young girls and women, who wanted to be able to run sometimes, so styles for them became very simple and natural again, while elder women continued to wear the heavy heads.

In a play called *The Rivals*, written in 1775, the author, Mr. Sheridan, shows us pretty young women elaborately dressed but with simple hairstyles, whereas an extraordinary old lady, called Mrs. Malaprop is still wearing an enormous wig and fantastic very large hats.

Another influence which caused hairstyles to become much simpler came from France. By the 1780s there was a lot of discontent in that country, because most of the people were very poor and almost starving, while a very few were very rich. Thinking people began to fear that a civil war might occur, and writers like Jean-Jacques Rousseau did what they could to encourage people to live simpler lives and to help the poor in every possible way.

Some of the people connected with King Louis XVI and his Queen continued the selfish ways they were accustomed to, and you have perhaps heard that when the Queen, Marie-Antoinette, heard that the people of Paris were starving and had no bread, she is supposed to have replied, 'Let them eat cake'. We do not know whether she actually said such a stupid and cruel thing, but she certainly behaved in that way. It is not surprising that things got worse until people's feelings got the better of them and they revolted, and the King and Queen and many of their court were executed.

This French Revolution had a great effect upon the ways that people dressed, even in England, and styles became much simpler. An untidy hairstyle, nicknamed the 'hedgehog' was popular for women for a time, as it was for men, perhaps because it showed that you were sympathetic with the revolutionaries, who certainly had no time to attend to their hair. A 'Brutus' cut was fashionable after the revolution, for women as it was for men—a shaggy uneven cut with an untidy fringe.

At this time, when English ladies were looking round for new ideas in clothes and hairdressing, they had their hair cut very very short, like the busts of ancient Greek and Roman godesses and empresses. Often this hairstyle was worn with a ribbon, or jewels or laurel leaves circling the head. One horrid style was called 'victim's hair'. This was an uneven cut, done to look like the hastily cut hair of the victims who were executed on the guillotine. For a short time some smart people wore a narrow red ribbon tied round their necks with this hairstyle, to make it seem as if they really were 'victims', but this unpleasant fashion did not last long.

Until the end of the eighteenth century, ladies had only known of a new fashion by seeing it worn, or hearing about it from an acquaintance or from seeing one of the fashion dolls which were sent regularly to England from Paris. Now, however, the new illustrated fashion magazines, such as the *Ladies' Magazine* and the *London Magazine* began to give several pages to showing new hairstyles.

Ladies carried masks when they went out of doors, to protect their complexions against cold in winter and against sunburn in summer. Face patches continued to be popular until the time of the French Revolution. In antique shops nowadays you can sometimes see lovely little patch boxes made of ivory, tortoiseshell, gold, silver or painted china, which were used by eighteenth-century ladies. They also used very delicate little china pots for their rouge.

Face powder was made of rice powder mixed with ground orris root. All kinds of cream and toilet waters were used, but people did not like to use plain water and soap, and were still dirty. One of the toilet waters which you can still buy today was first made in the eighteenth century by a perfumer working in Cologne, in Germany. Do you know its name, and why it was called this? The date on each bottle tells us when it was first made.

The 'hedgehog' style

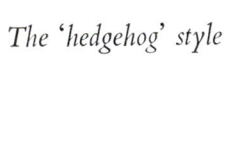

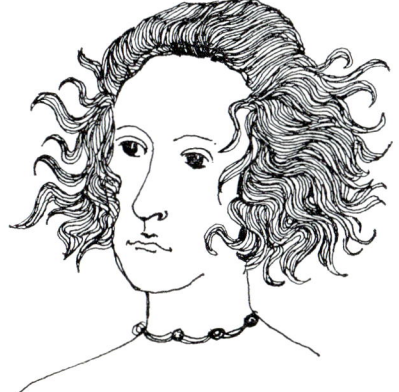

CHAPTER FIVE

Styles for men and boys 1800 - 1914

At the beginning of the nineteenth century the smartest men from all European countries had their clothes tailored in London, just as they do nowadays. Before then, Paris had been the fashion centre, but the dangerous conditions there during the French Revolution drove customers away, and most of them did not go back.

There was a small group of very smart men, called 'dandies', who led fashions in dress and in hairstyles, just as the 'macaronis' had done in the eighteenth century. Two of the leading dandies were the Prince Regent, later King George IV, and a Mr. George Brummell, known as 'Beau Brummell' because he looked so handsome and dressed so splendidly. He had a great influence on men's fashions and many people began to copy his habit of washing himself regularly and wearing clean underclothes. This was something quite new and from this time onwards Englishmen paid more attention to personal cleanliness than they had done before.

Beau Brummell wore a mass of curls at his temples and over his forehead. It is said that he found he needed three hairdressers to arrange his hair: one for the front curls, another for the side curls and another for the back of his head. This may not be true, but it is certain that any man wanting to be

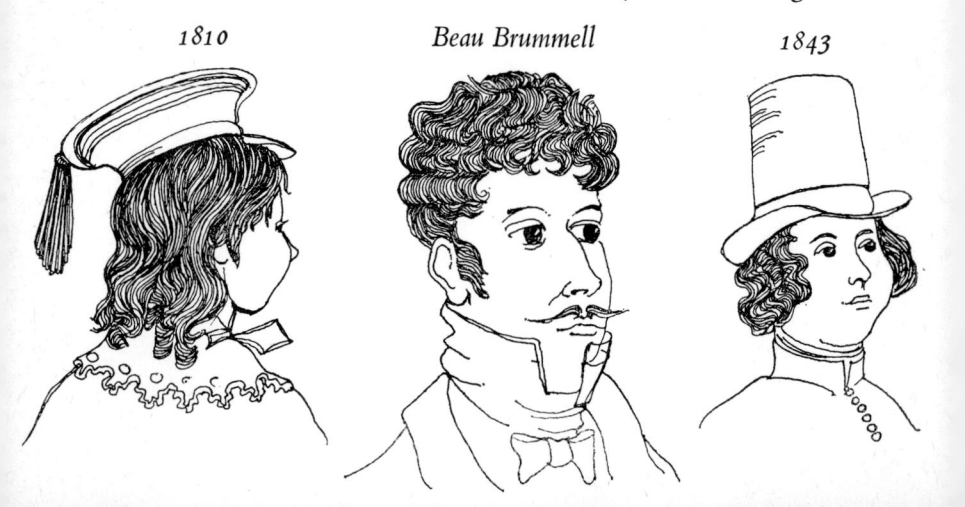

1810 *Beau Brummell* *1843*

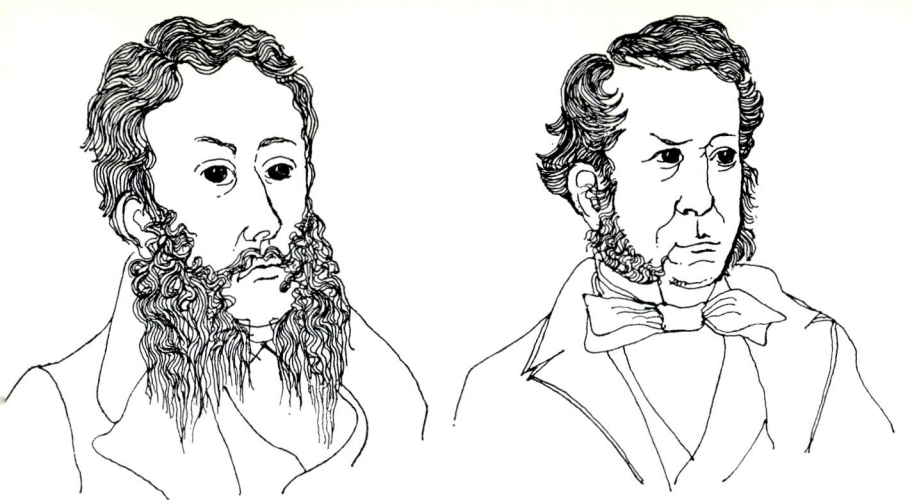

'Piccadilly weapers'   *Side whiskers*

fashionable at this time had to use curling irons and to take a lot of time and trouble in doing his hair.

    Men no longer wore wigs unless they were very old, and natural hair worn shorter was fashionable throughout the whole of the nineteenth century. Very high collars were worn, and so for the sake of comfort men had their hair cut short at the back, but in the front they wore curls, fringes and waves, at various times. Side hair was brushed forward over the cheeks in Regency times and from then onwards long side-pieces gradually came into fashion.

    In the 1850s whiskers and moustaches became fashionable and a fashion for wearing a beard grew as a result of the Crimean War. You will probably have seen pictures of Florence Nightingale nursing soldiers who had been fighting against the Russians in the Crimea, and you may have heard the poem 'The Charge of the Light Brigade'. Officers in the Crimea wore beards, probably because they had no time to shave during the fighting, and were very short of water. When they returned to England after the war, fashionable men thought the style looked attractive and copied it.

    Long side whiskers, called 'Piccadilly weapers' or 'Dundreary whiskers', named after a character in a popular play, were worn with beards and, later on, without them. After about 1870 smaller, neater whiskers were worn and by the end of the century heavy 'cavalry' moustaches were popular.

    As men gradually began to pay more attention to having clean bodies and fresh-smelling clothes, they began to use perfumed soap and even toilet waters, though this was not general until much more recently. Charles Dickens, the writer, when he wrote *Bleak House* in 1853, described a young man who was evidently taking great pains about his looks:

> He had on an entirely new suit of glossy clothes, a shiny hat, black kid gloves, a neckerchief (scarf) of a variety of colours, a large hothouse flower in his button-hole, and a thick gold ring upon his little finger. Besides which he quite scented the dining room with bear's grease and other perfumery.

One of the items of perfumery that the young man used would probably have been hair oil. Whether your hair was worn in curls or waves, or straight, you liked to have it well oiled, to keep it sleek. A special kind of oil was imported from Macassar for use on the hair and many wives and mothers found that their chairs were being ruined by the marks left on the backs when their husbands and sons leaned their heads against them. So a fashion began for hanging coloured or embroidered cloths over the backs of armchairs. These were called anti-macassars. 'Anti' is Latin for 'against'; another word formed in the same way is 'antiseptic'. See if you can find others.

In 1886 a book appeared which became so popular that it had an influence on boys' clothes and hair styles. This was *Little Lord Fauntleroy* by Mrs Hodgson Burnett. The illustrations showed the 'Little Lord' in a velvet suit, with a lace collar, a large-brimmed hat with a feather and long hair. Many boys whose mothers dressed them in this fancy style must have secretly hated the author and illustrator of the book.

At the beginning of our century men began to wear their hair with a side parting, instead of the centre parting which had been so popular for a long time. A clean-shaven face became popular, but less and less attention was paid to differing hairstyles. It was thought 'unmanly' to pay much attention to your hair and it was worn short and neat.

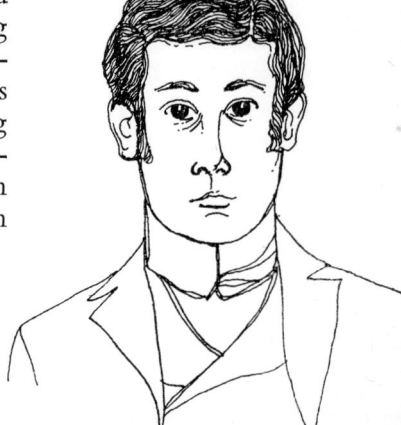

36   *Early twentieth century*

CHAPTER SIX

Styles for women and girls 1800 - 1914

In the early years of the nineteenth century, during what was called the Regency Period, after the Prince Regent, ladies either wore their hair very short and straight, or else piled up in a chignon or topknot, with curls at the sides. Between 1805 and 1810 there was a rage for one-sided effects in hairdressing, with each side of the hair done differently—flat on one side and with a cluster of curls on the other.

It was fashionable to show your ears at this time, so earrings became popular. So did elaborate jewelled combs to wear in your hair and gold wreaths of laurel leaves. One particularly popular hair ornament was a long gold hairpin, five or six inches long, in the form of an arrow.

Artificial flowers were also worn in the hair and a prosperous trade in these started in France. Previously the only artificial flowers made were roses, made in Italy for decorating churches, but not for fashion purposes.

In Regency times very pale colours were fashionable for women's clothes, so make-up was pale too. Heavy, elaborate make-up was too much a reminder of the aristocrats in France before the Revolution, and therefore not popular. Rice powder was used, and Eau de Cologne, and soap. You made your own cosmetics at home unless you were very rich. Your toilet

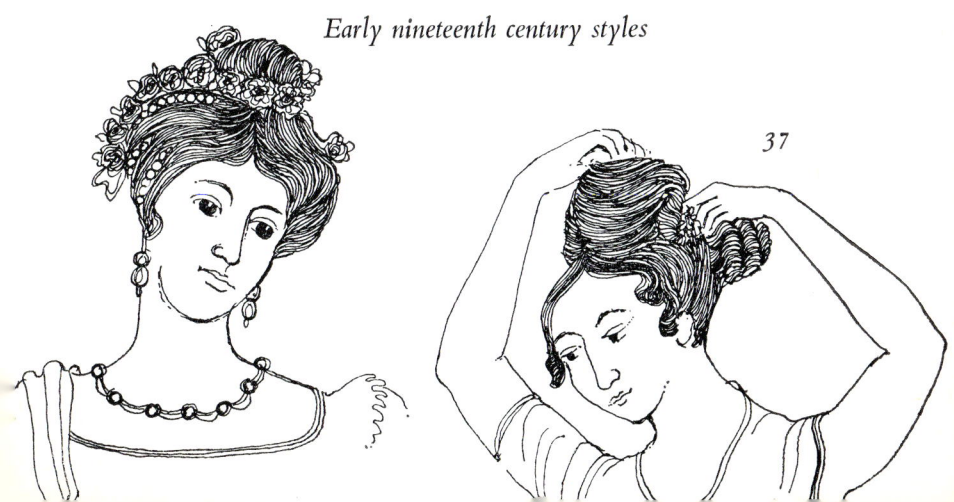

Early nineteenth century styles

1825   *1843*

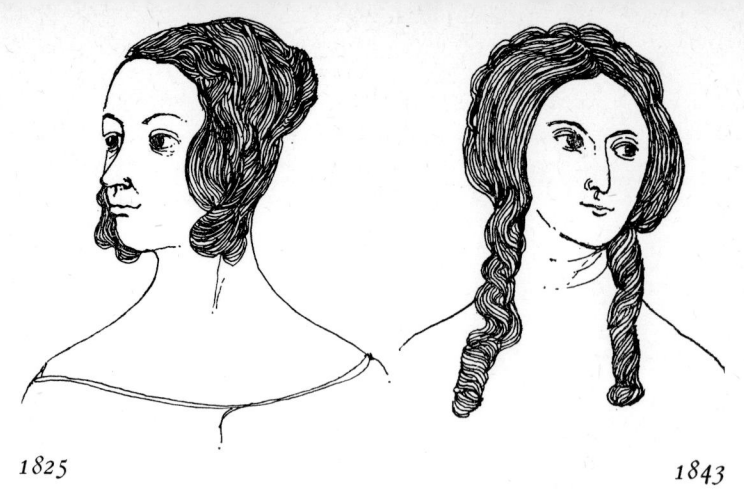

water you would make from a mixture of glycerine and rose-water; you used lampblack for mascara; and you rubbed your cheeks to make them pink. You did not say you were going to 'make up'. You were going to 'rouge and pearl'.

From about 1835 hairstyles, like fashions, began to change more quickly. Perhaps this was because many people were prosperous because of the new factories and coalfields being developed. People were getting about more and had more opportunities to see how others dressed, and to copy new styles. At this time it was very elegant to wear your hair in 'Apollo's knots'. These were loops of tightly plaited hair, fixed with ribbons, strings of beads, long pins or carved combs. False curls and switches of hair were much used and it was very smart to dye your hair.

A 'ferronière' was a fine chain, or a velvet ribbon worn round your head, with a jewel or medallion in the middle of your forehead.

By 1840 a new, sleeker style was fashionable. You too used macassar oil to smooth your hair on either side of a centre parting; and you pulled it back into a chignon or 'bun', low at the back of your neck. You kept your chignon in place with a large ornamental ivory or tortoiseshell comb, or with large hairpins. For grand evening occasions married women wore flowers, lace, plumes and jewellery in their hair. Young unmarried girls usually wore their heads without any decoration.

Waving the hair at the side of your head was very new in the 1850s. Nobody had yet thought of permanent waving, so you had to use little iron tongs which you heated over the fire. In the 1860s it became fashionable to wear a little cushion made

A chignon

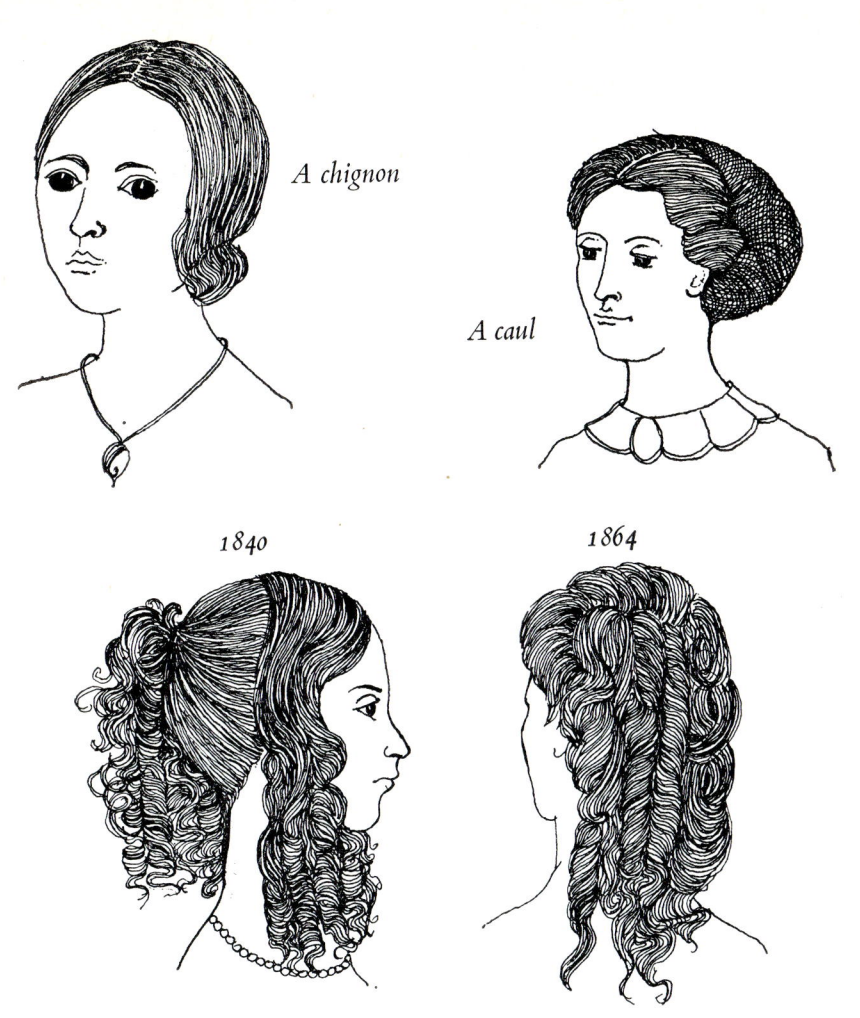

A caul

1840   *1864*

of horsehair to raise the height of your coiffure, instead of having it flat on top. Sometimes ladies wore pads at the back too, to give greater bulk to the chignon, which in time got bigger and bigger.

A 'caul' now became necessary to keep your hair in place. This was called a 'net' later on. In the 1850s it was of braided silk and velvet ribbon, fastened with gilt buckles and buttons. Or you might have preferred to ask your hairdresser to make you a net of your own hair when it was cut, so that it was invisible.

In the 1870s it was no longer smart to have your hair oiled and sleek. You tried to look rather untidy, with rolls of hair, ringlets, braids and bands.

A 'waterfall'

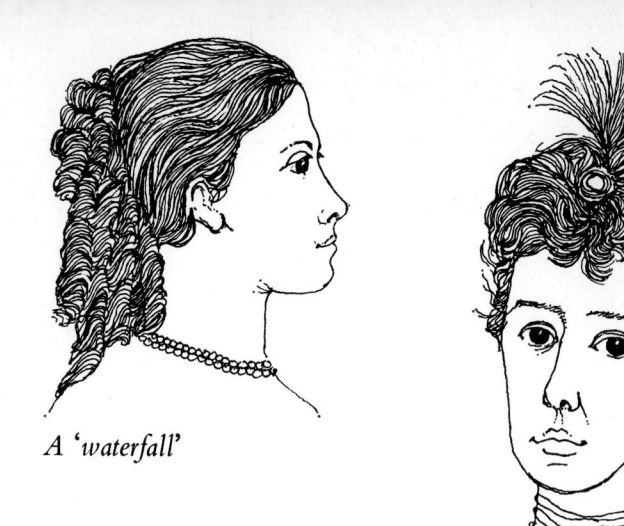

Lily Langtry

The most elaborate fashion at this time was the 'waterfall'. This was a style in which you had heavy curls cascading down your back and fixed into a kind of long roll, so you can see where the name came from. Sometimes this back hair was enclosed in a large net and sometimes not, but nearly always it meant that you had to pad out your hair with false pieces. Often the front of your hair was cut short and worn in 'bangs' or whisps, rather like a thin fringe. Curling tongs were even used on little girls' hair because of the new craze for curls. Round combs covered with silk or velvet material were worn over your head from ear to ear to hold your hair in place. After 1865, when *Alice in Wonderland* was first published, an 'Alice band' was very popular.

No respectable lady used any make-up at this time and certainly must never do anything in public to improve her appearance. Queen Victoria had very strict views and her influence spread to all kinds of people; it was fashionable to be prim and to despise the free and easy behaviour of eighteenth-century and Regency ladies. You would steam your face at home over a basin of hot water, use soap to clean your skin and cold cream at night, but nothing more.

In the 1870s it was very smart to have red hair. In a book called *The Art of Beauty: a Book for Women and Girls*, published in 1878, the author suggested that it was the Pre-Raphaelite painters, Burne-Jones, Millais and their friends Watts and William Morris who encouraged this fashion, and added: 'Red hair—once to say a woman had red hair was social assassination—now it is the rage'.

In the 1880s you wore your hair in a bun on the top of your head, and no longer at the back of your neck. You had a curled fringe over your forehead and tiny ringlets over your ears and when you wore a bonnet on top of this hair-do you looked very much like a lady of the end of the seventeenth century, wearing her fontange. Turn to page 19 and compare.

Whenever curls and ringlets were in fashion, ladies whose hair was straight had to use false curls, for there was no safe way of curling natural hair, though false hair could be curled. In 1890 a Frenchman, Monsieur Marcel began to use a pair of pointed tongs, which he heated and, with a twist of his wrist he was able to make waves which lasted a few days. This method of 'marcel waving' spread throughout Europe.

Until the nineteenth century fashions in women's dress and hairstyles had nearly always been set by royalty, but now actresses began to have an important influence. The Queen was not smart and did not approve of high fashion, but there were famous actresses who did. The most famous of these was Lily Langtry, said to be one of the most beautiful women in the world. She wore her hair waved and with a low chignon, and this became the rage. She was a blonde, and because of this fair hair was fashionable until the turn of the century. Incidentally Lily Langtry had an important influence on dress

Monsieur Marcel with a customer in 1922

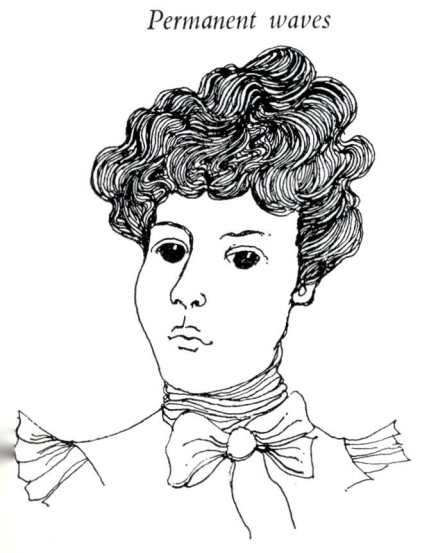

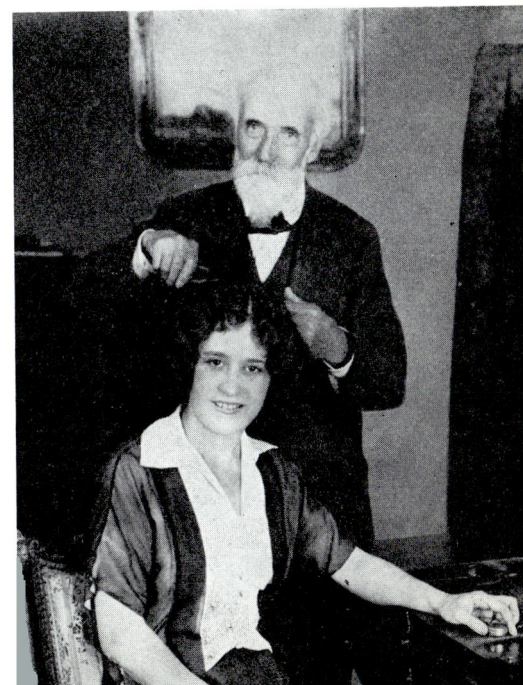

Permanent waves

too. She lived in Jersey, was called 'The Jersey Lily' and had noticed the long-sleeved knitted garments which the island fishermen wore. She had one made for her and liked it so much that she ordered others and before long fashionable women in England and in France began to wear 'jerseys'—as a great many men and women and boys and girls have done ever since.

Topknots, chignons, braids, switches and clusters of curls were all in fashion at the beginning of our century. It was smart to make your head look 'big', which meant that you fluffed your hair out as much as possible with your comb. You kept a little kind of bag, called a 'hair tidy' hanging on your dressing table and collected the combings that came out of your hair; and when you had enough you would have them made into a pad to fill out the puffs of your hairstyle. This is how a lady who was a leader of fashion at the beginning of our century, describes the style she remembers when she was young:

> Hair was first tied in bunches with little bits of tape and then pinned up in puffs and mounds and curls attached to long wires fixed on at the side. At least twenty minutes a day must be devoted to brushing it. When it was cut it had to be singed with a taper, otherwise it would split and bleed.[1]

The fluffy kind of hairstyle came to an end when 'electrical' waving was first used in 1906. A Mr Karl Nessler, a German hairdresser in London invented this new way of waving hair, but it was very expensive and took between eight and twelve hours to do! It is not surprising that only very few women were willing to have their hair waved in this new way, but after a few years it became quicker and cheaper, and popular as 'Nestlé Permanent Waving'. The craze for blonde hair died out when Lily Langtry retired from the stage and an auburn colour again became popular. This was produced by using the liquid from soaking the leaves of the henna bush, which grows in certain parts of Africa and the East. Dyeing your hair was now thought quite a respectable thing to do, even in quite strict families.

[1] From *Grace and Favour* by Loelia, Duchess of Westminster.

Make-up was beginning to be respectable too. Tiny powder boxes of gold or silver were carried in a smart lady's handbag; compact powders were made; vanishing creams were new; but you never dreamed of putting on any of these 'beautifiers' anywhere except in private. It was at Selfridges' store when it opened in London in 1911, that cosmetics were first sold openly instead of from under the counter. Until then, respectable women were still shy of being seen buying cosmetics and perfumes.

The elaborate hairstyles worn by fashionable women before the First World War meant that hairdressers had to be very skilled in making up artificial hair. Most of the hair came from abroad, and there were hair dealers who toured parts of England and bought the locks of country women and girls. Sometimes these men were very dishonest; they would knock on a cottage door, and if the occupier had a fine head of hair he would offer her a pound or so for it; then he would snip off all he could, and rush off without paying anything! After a time there was such a fuss made about the unfair ways of collecting hair, that the practice died out.

A hairdresser's advertisement 1905

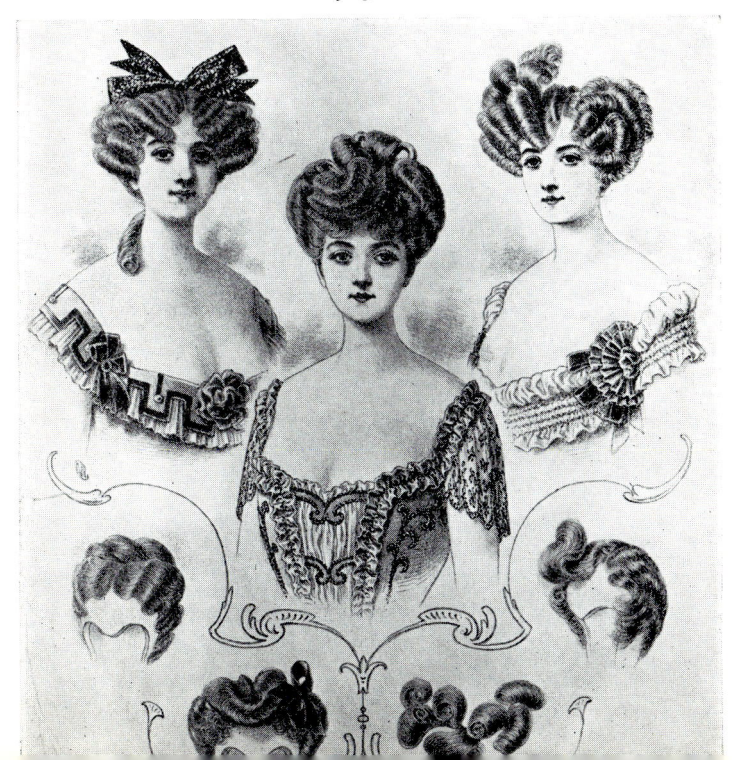

CHAPTER SEVEN

Hairstyles since the Great War

Wars and revolutions have always had an effect on people's dress and their hairstyles, as well as on their behaviour. We have seen that both the Civil War in England in the seventeenth century and the Revolution in France in the eighteenth century led to changes in hairstyles.

The same thing happened after the Great War of 1914–18, and the Second World War of 1939–45. During both these wars most women did some kind of work outside the home, even if they had never done so before, so their clothes had to be practical and their hairstyles very simple. Men's styles did not change so much.

Long hair was a nuisance if you were working in a factory, and it was dangerous too. So between 1914 and 1918 some women had their long hair cut off and wore it in a 'bob'. There was a great fuss about this at first and many people thought it was not decent for women to have such short hair. The new style was not at all general until the 1920s, when many schoolgirls had their hair bobbed and wore it decorated with a large bow of black ribbon.

Suzanne Lenglen, a famous French tennis player, won the women's singles championship at Wimbledon in 1923 and started a new hair fashion. She wore a band round her bobbed hair during the match, low down over her forehead, to keep the hair out of her eyes, and this started a craze for wearing what was called 'headache' bands. You can see these on the girls in the early films that are shown sometimes.

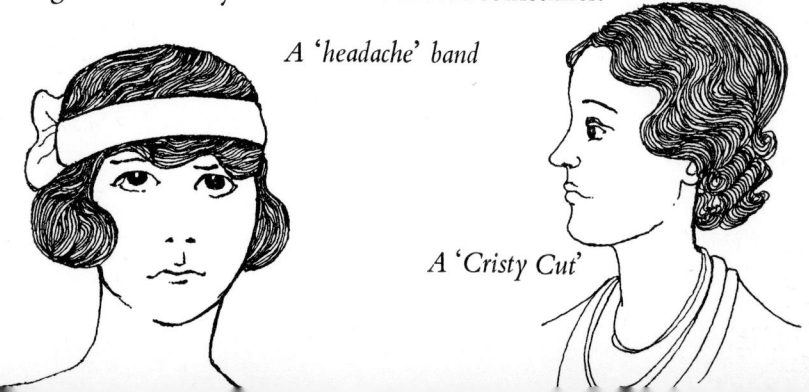

A 'headache' band

A 'Cristy Cut'

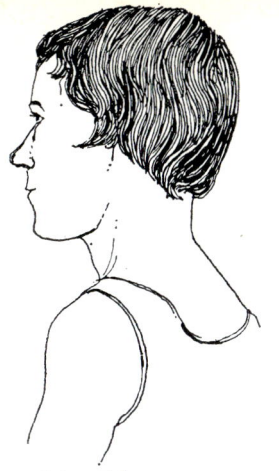

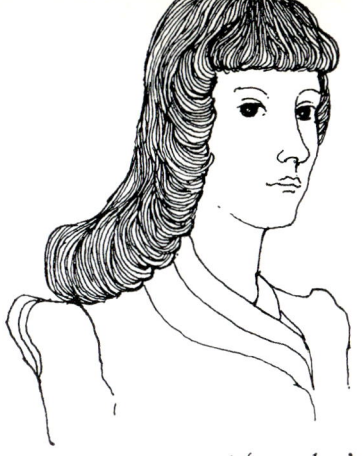

A 'shingle'   *A 'page boy'*

Shorter hair meant that ordinary people could have smarter hairstyles. The elaborate styles of before the war had been very expensive to keep up and were only suitable for people who had plenty of servants, and plenty of time. Shampoos began to be used instead of soap, and many kinds were made and sold quite cheaply. But some people thought that shampoos were dangerous, particularly after the death of a lady in the hairdressing department of a famous London shop in July 1909. She died from fumes given off by a dry shampoo and for several months it looked as if the hairdressing business would suffer, but the scare died out.

Soon after the bob, hair began to be worn even shorter. In 1924 the 'shingle' and soon afterwards the 'Eton crop' were very mannish styles which many people objected to, but which went very well with the very straight, shapeless short dresses of the twenties. These short hairstyles were all worn straight, not curled or waved.

By 1930 shoulder-length hair had begun to look smart and 'upswept' styles were worn with the new, longer dresses. In 1935 'coronation' curls were very smart, worn over your forehead and with the side hair swept up. Do you know whose coronation gave the name to this new style? In 1937 a 'page boy' set, with the ends curled under, which was like the style worn by a page in the Middle Ages, began a new interest in smooth, straight hair which has lasted ever since.

'Machineless' waving began to be advertised in the middle 1930s and a few years later the 'Cristy Cut' was introduced from America, named after a hairdresser who found a way of encouraging hair to wave by a special way of cutting. Chemical ways of 'perming' hair developed more and more during this time.

From the 1920s onwards, the cinema began to have a great influence on what women wore and on how they did their hair. Film stars were glamorous and many women and girls copied their hairstyles as nearly as possible. A fashion for altering your hair colour and for wearing a light platinum 'streak' began when a platinum blonde actress, Jean Harlow, became popular a few years before the 1939 war. Before then you did not dye your hair unless you were going grey and wanted to pretend you weren't, and so of course you kept the matter very secret. From the middle thirties, however, it was smart to tint your hair blue or violet—though not with powder as they did in the eighteenth century.

During the last war 'snoods' were worn a great deal by women doing factory work and others who did not have much time to bother with complicated hairdos. The snood was rather like the caul of the 1850s.

In the twenties and thirties there was no general hairstyle for men. Most of them wore it smooth and oiled, and brushed straight back from the forehead, without a parting. In the hairdressing trade journals of the mid-thirties, permanent waving was suggested for men, but this did not become popular. Some men wore moustaches and a few wore beards, but the majority were clean shaven.

After the 1939–45 war men seemed to want a change from the very short haircuts which they had to have in the Services, and they began to wear their hair longer on top, with 'full back and sides'. This continued during the fifties and nowadays long hair is worn by so many young men that it may be that we are gradually moving towards a time when all men will wear long hair or long wigs again. Medieval bobs and fringes are already worn, and the 'Teddy Boy' styles of the 1950s, called after the Edwardian fashions of the beginning of this century, no longer seem so ridiculous as they did a few years ago.

More and more women began to go to beauty shops between the two wars, to have their hair trimmed, shampooed and set into waves with a new plastic lotion, and they now began to use make-up even in public. So many cosmetics were on the market that it became necessary to pass laws to make sure that harmful ingredients are not used.

Late in the 1920s it became smart for those who could afford it, to spend their summer holidays in the South of France and to come home with a 'sun tan'. This was quite a new idea, for until that time it was only labourers and farmers and other people who worked in the open air who had brown skins. Wealthy women had previously spent a great deal of money and time in protecting their skin *against* the sun, and it had been smart to look pale and delicate. Special oils and lotions to deepen your tan began to appear in the 1930s and brownish face powders were produced for the first time. Since the last war, nearly everyone has thought it attractive and smart to have a sunburnt skin.

Another big change during this century has been the use of deodorants. Ladies used to wear cotton dress-shields or dress-preservers, sewn inside their garments under the arms, for no chemical perspiration checks were known until recent years. It seems that our ancestors did not consider the smell of perspiration to be unattractive, as we all do nowadays; perhaps that was because nobody knew how to avoid it. Nowadays it is a rare person—man or woman, boy or girl—who does not prefer to use a deodorant regularly, and so make sure that they do not smell nasty to other people.

Keith West 1967 *Cilla Black 1967*

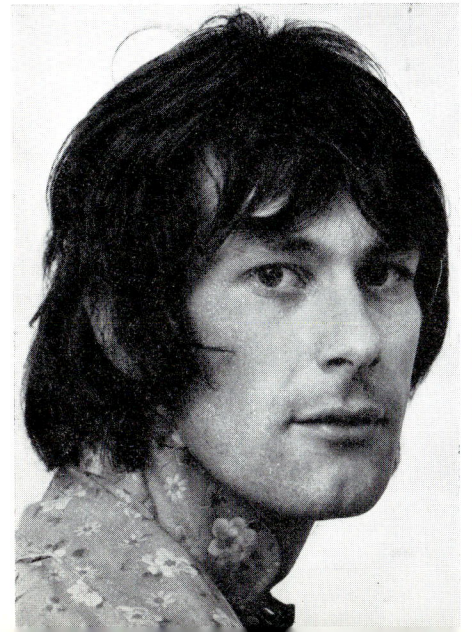

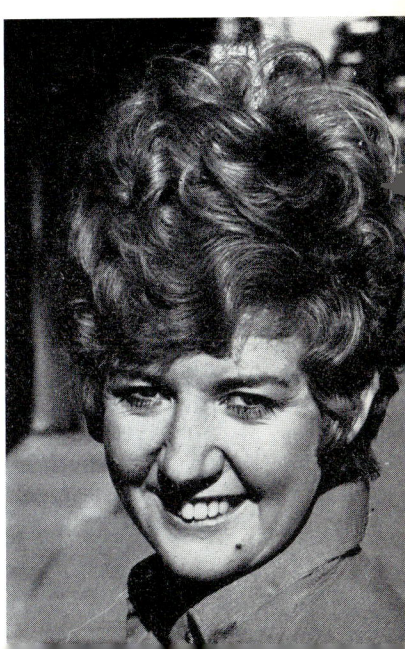

CHAPTER EIGHT

How do we know?

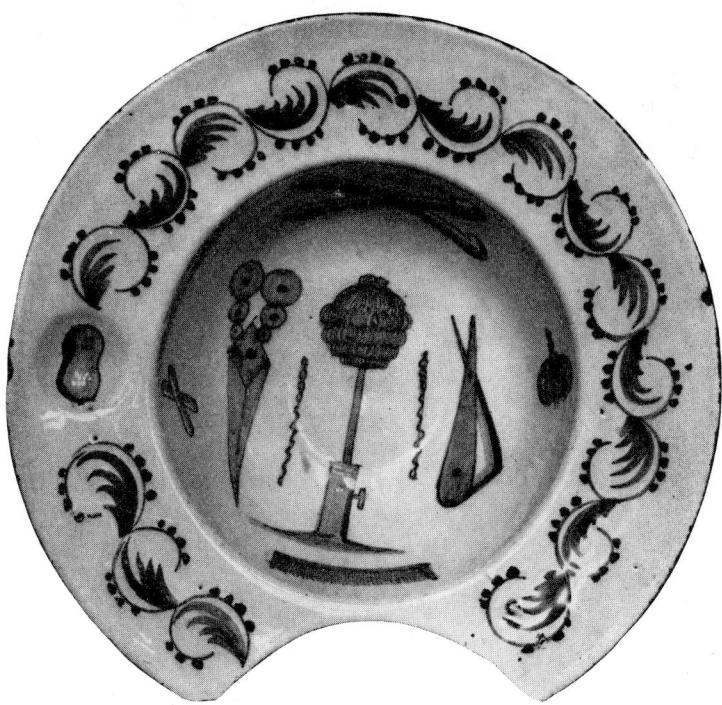

Here is a plate which was used in a barber's shop in about 1700. It is in the museum at Brighton and you can see that it is decorated with various barber's tools and a wig on an adjustable stand.

Am I imagining these facts about this old plate, or making them up? If not, how do I know its date? its use? its meaning?

This is a complicated business, because there are many answers. In the Brighton Museum the plate is labelled 'Barber's plate of Lambeth Ware, *c.* 1700' (*c.* means 'about', from the Latin word 'circa'), and because the Curator there is a responsible, knowledgeable man, I tend to believe what he says about the plate. But how does *he* know? It would not be impossible for him to be wrong; experts do make mistakes sometimes, and anyway what one expert says may differ from what another says. No, we need to know how our friend the Curator of the Brighton Museum decided what to put on his label.

Luckily, human beings always leave a lot of things behind them when they die, and many of these things tell us about the owners. You have probably seen photographs of your parents when they were little, and of your grandparents; perhaps even of *their* parents too. Perhaps you have an old photograph with a name and a date on the back. If so, that photograph is an important piece of evidence, and tells how people like your grandmother or great-grandmother dressed in the year it was taken.

But photography was not known until the 1840s, so no photograph can tell us anything about a period earlier than that. What other kind of evidence—about clothes, hairstyles, furniture, or any other daily matters, can we look for? Before the 1840s, if parents wanted to have a record of what their children looked like at a certain age, they had them drawn, or painted by an artist. If they were wealthy they chose a well-known portrait painter and had to pay a high fee; but ordinary people sometimes had their portraits painted, too, by somebody less expensive, or by an artist who wanted to have some practice, and didn't charge at all. Often the artist painted the name of the 'sitter', and his own name and the date, at the bottom of the picture. Look at the painting below and see what it tells you about the fashions in dress and hairstyles of the year 1620.

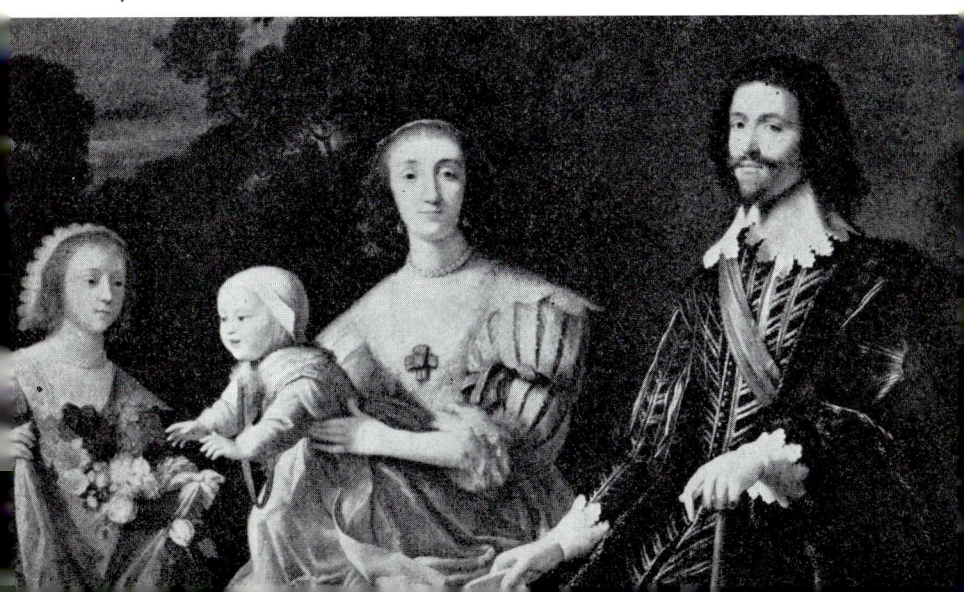

Other 'picture' evidence can be found on early tombs too. In the Middle Ages the person buried was shown in a drawing on brass over the place where he was buried, and later on stone statues were put on the tops of tombs. These show us the kind of clothes the dead person had worn, though the details are often less easy to see than they are when we look at a large painting.

These, and other picture ways of discovering how our ancestors dressed and did their hair, are not the only clues we can find. People don't only leave pictures behind them, they often leave writings too. Letters, diaries, wills, Church and Town Hall registers, even School registers and log-books can tell us very interesting facts about the people who wrote them, or those about whom they are written. Here are a few of the entries in the family account book of the Duke of Bedford in the seventeenth century:

May 1653	For tape, for black ribbon, for two fine ivory combs for the children, of the pedlar	7s	0d
April 1654	To a barber for trimming Mr Edward and Mr Robert	2s	0d
April 1661	(for the Coronation of King Charles II). For silk and worsted stockings, shoes, gloves, half-shirts, bands and band-strongs, hats and feathers for the pages and footmen	£35 8s	10d
July 1670	To Mr Freiston for two periwigs for my lady's page	£2 0s	0d
Nov. 1681	To the page, for twice cutting his hair	1s	0d

A needlework picture of a Stuart lady

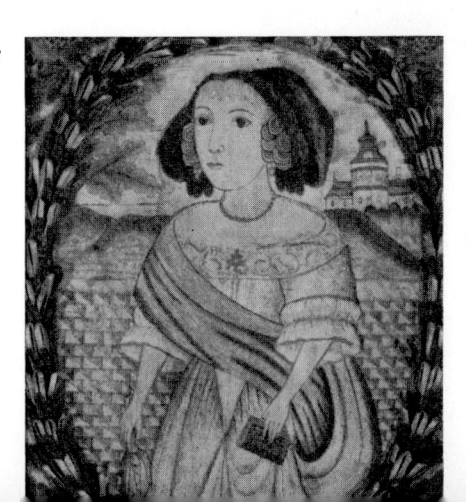

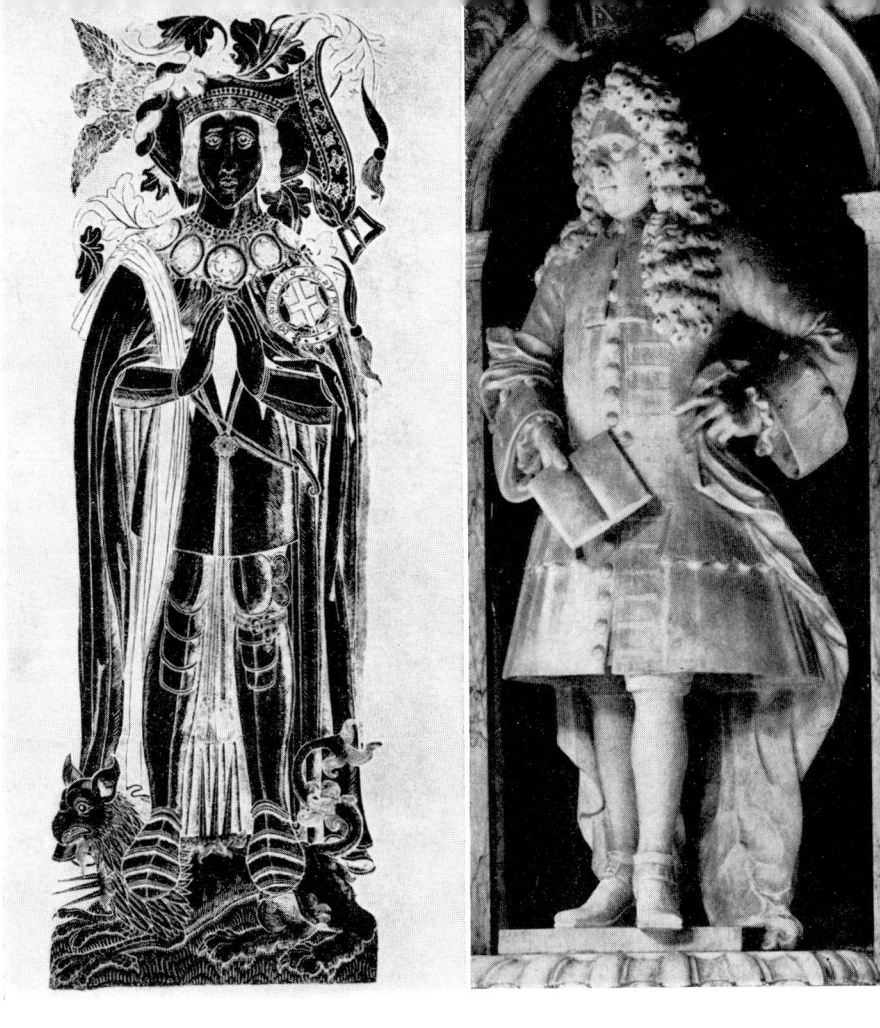

Three more types of 'picture' evidence:

a rubbing from a brass of 1538

a statue of 1714

a drawing in a 14th century manuscript

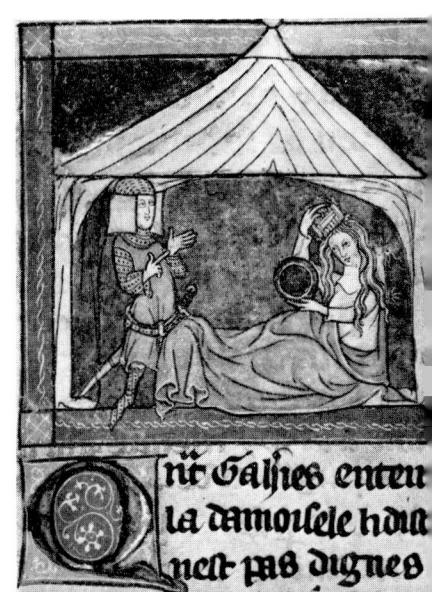

Of course stories can tell us a good deal about the time of the *writer*—even if he has decided to write his plot about some far distant and imaginary time. Buildings, too, are full of clues about the past, and the furniture and curtains, the silver and china and cooking pots and weapons that were used long ago all have a story to tell, if we look carefully and know what to look for.

That is the important thing—knowing where to begin, getting our eyes tuned up. I am always surprised that some boys know so much about the shapes of aeroplanes, and that my daughters and their friends know so many pop tunes and who sings them. I myself don't know nearly as much about either aeroplanes or pop tunes, but I know that, if I wanted to, I could learn about them by looking, by listening, and by talking things over. It is familiarity and enthusiasm which can start us off on finding interesting clues in things that, at first, we know nothing about.

So, going back to the barber's plate on page 48, I feel sure that the date 'c. 1700' is right, not merely because I trust the expert, but because I have seen a lot of paintings of gentlemen of that time wearing wigs like that one. And if I knew more than I do about earthenware and china I would, by handling the plate, be able to say that it was made in a way that is known to have been fashionable in pottery workshops in Lambeth, south of London, in the late seventeenth and early eighteenth centuries.

Detective work of this kind is absolutely fascinating, and one of the exciting things about going to a strange district is to look around you and 'date' the buildings, find out why the streets have the names they have, and so on.

Similarly, when visiting museums and art galleries and large country houses you may perhaps be able to find out more about hairstyles in the past, and to check the information I have written in this book.

CHAPTER NINE

Hairdressing as a career

There is hardly anybody who has not been to the hairdresser's at some time or another. You yourself have had your hair cut more often than you can remember, and perhaps you have had it shampooed in a salon sometimes as well. You may even have wondered what it is like to be a hairdresser, and perhaps you have thought of becoming one yourself.

What would it be like?

Being a hairdresser can be a very happy and satisfying job if you are the right type of person for it. The work is varied and interesting and, of course, very useful. To be a good hairdresser you must be clever with your hands and you must have a good 'eye': that is, you need to be able to judge how things look, and whether, for example, this or that style or colour of hair suits a particular customer's shape of face and head. It is very important that a hairdresser shall like people and be able to get on well with them. A pleasant manner counts a lot, for if you start off by disliking your customers and being disagreeable or rude to them you will never make a success of the job, and they will soon decide to go somewhere else where the assistants are friendly.

You must not be afraid of hard work if you want to be a hairdresser. There is a great deal to learn and there are always hectic days, when there seem to be too many customers and not enough time or energy with which to get things done. You need to be able to work in a team and fit in with people of all kinds. It is important to be an adaptable kind of person, because you can never be sure what may happen next in a hairdresser's, and a sense of fun is a great help there, as it is everywhere else. You must be fit and strong, for the hours are long and the work is often strenuous. You are on your feet for most of the time and it is tiring to work in a hot atmosphere. A good deal of any hairdresser's work is in steamy surroundings.

It is important to look ahead when you are deciding what

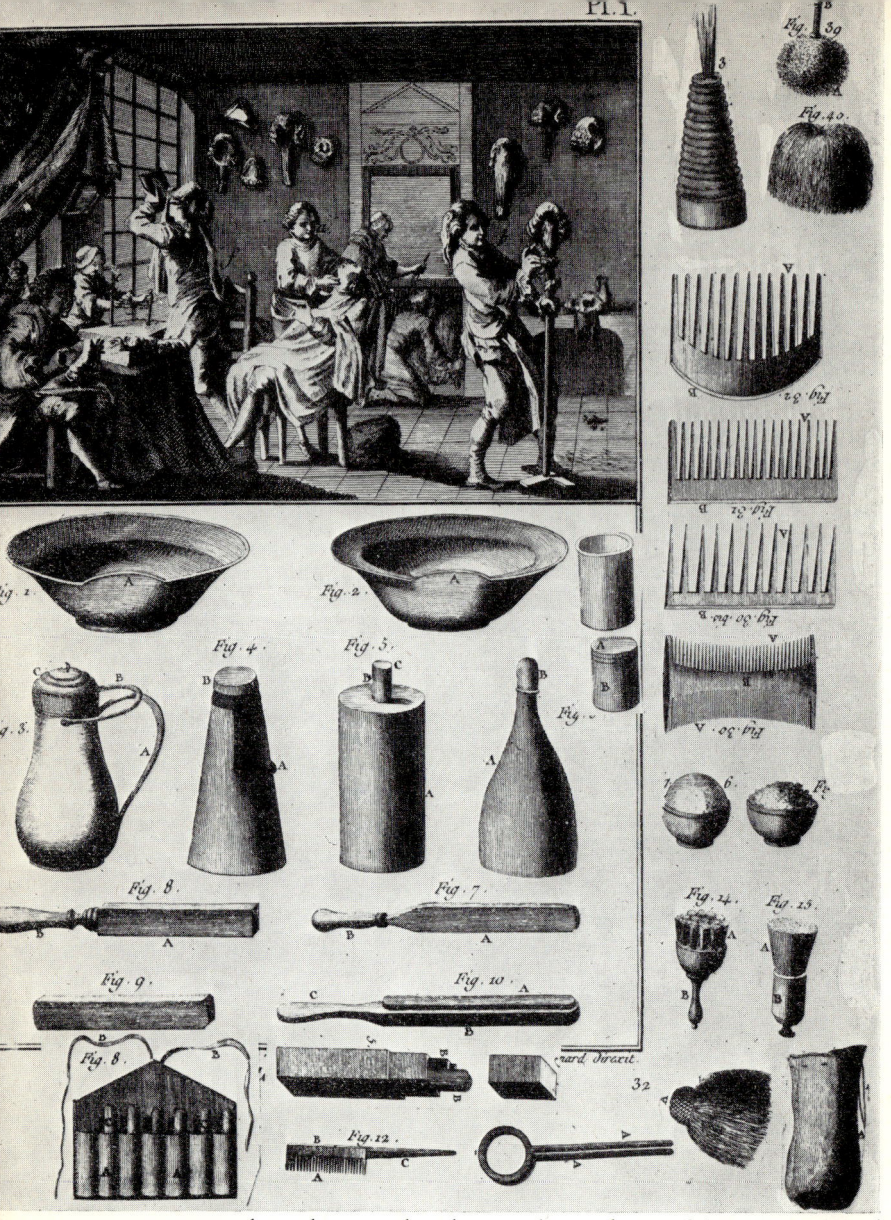

An eighteenth century hairdressing shop and some of the equipment used

job you want to take up. Usually jobs that are well paid at the beginning are those in which you cannot get promotion and earn much more later on. And in any case, if you are sensible, you will want to learn a *skill* that you can use in the future and which you can feel is a special part of *you*.

It is just as important for a girl to look ahead like this as it is for a boy, because you may find that you have to work after you get married, or you may want to do so. None of us can ever be sure what we shall have to do in the future, or where we shall be living. Prospects in hairdressing are very good and it is work that you can do part-time later on, if need be, and also something that you can do in any city in the world. There are very few jobs that are so flexible—except being a nurse, a doctor, a dentist or a teacher—and if you are thinking of any of those you will probably not be reading this chapter.

You won't earn a lot of money at first as a hairdresser, but that is not the most important thing. You will be paid a wage while you are training and how much you earn after that depends a good deal on you and on the sort of salon you choose to work in. The minimum wages are fixed by law, but many employers pay more than the minimum to somebody whom they like and whose work brings in a lot of customers. And you will get tips if you are pleasant and helpful and look after customers well. If you are living at home you will be able to manage during your training period, but perhaps your parents can help you a little with overalls and so on.

The most satisfying thing about a job in hairdressing and beauty culture is that you are all the time helping people. You help them to make the most of their appearance and to take care of themselves. Every customer who goes out of the hairdresser's feels better than when he or she came in, and you can feel pleased and proud that you have brought that about.

Girls, of course, go in for ladies hairdressing and beauty culture, but boys can choose to work in either ladies' or gentlemen's salons, and it is quite a good idea for a boy to take up both.

If you are a rather independent and ambitious kind of person you may like to look ahead to a time when you could have a hairdresser's business of your own. This could be great fun and a real challenge, but it is not something that you could hope to do until you have had several years' experience—and have saved some money!

There are two ways of learning to be a hairdresser. You can become an apprentice or you can to go a Technical College.

1. *Apprenticeship* takes three years. You can begin when you are fifteen, but it is better to stay on at school and do some

more advanced work, and then start your apprenticeship between sixteen and eighteen.

Most employers give a special welcome to boys and girls who have stayed at school after they are fifteen, because they think they will be better able to take responsibility and to cope with the job. And if you do wait at least another year before leaving, you have given yourself time to think over carefully and to discuss what you would like to do.

First you must find a Master Hairdresser who will take you on as an apprentice, and it is very important to choose a good one. Don't of course, go to the first one you think of, or the one nearest to where you live. It isn't a good idea, either, to decide where you would like to take an apprenticeship by the colour of the curtains in the salon, or because there is a nice boy or girl working there whom you would like to get to know! There are plenty of other ways of making an acquaintance, and you may in the end decide that he or she isn't so special after all, but once you have signed on as an apprentice you are almost bound to stay there for the three years.

Ask one or two young people who are, or were, hairdressing apprentices whether their boss is kind and understanding and a good craftsman, and what the conditions are like. And perhaps your mother or father knows somebody who can give an opinion as to the best hairdresser to go to. A list of all the Master Hairdressers in your district who have vacancies for apprentices can be seen at your local Youth Employment Office.

The Government makes laws about apprentices and these are printed in a leaflet, issued by the Ministry of Labour, called 'Wages Regulations (Hairdressing) Order (34)', which has to be pinned up in the staff room of every hairdresser's. You could buy a copy if you wanted to, from the Stationery Office, York House, Kingsway, London, W.C.2, for 1s. 3d. You probably would not be able to understand much of it—I couldn't—but what it really says is how many hours hairdressing apprentices shall work, and what pay and holidays they shall have.

No employer is allowed to take on too many apprentices and the 'Order' gives instructions about that too. There must not be more than one apprentice to each trained hairdresser,

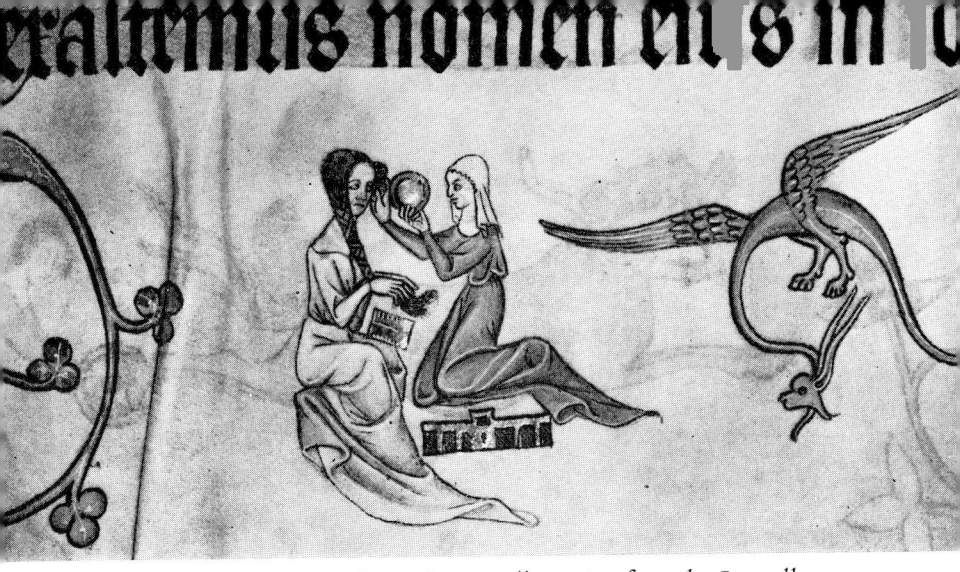

A twelfth century lady at her toilet—an illustration from the Luttrell Psalter

otherwise the apprentices might not get enough attention or be properly taught.

There is an organization called the National Apprenticeship Council for the Hairdressing Craft, and this also lays down rules to help hairdressers and their apprentices to work together happily. These rules are about such things as how apprentices are to be taught, and what they can be expected to do. So you can see that you will be well looked after if you decide to train to be a hairdresser, and no employer can behave unfairly, even if he wanted to.

When you decide to begin as a hairdressing apprentice you will be on trial for three months and after that you both have to sign what is called an 'Indenture'. This is an agreement between you and your employer and it has to be signed by your parent or guardian as well as by your employer and you, and also by a representative of the National Apprenticeship Council. (Head Office, 39 Grafton Way, London, W.1.) After the trial period, if all has gone well, you will go on learning and working with the same employer for the rest of the three years. If for any reason your employer cannot continue to train you—if, for example, he falls ill or dies, or has to move, the local representative of the National Apprenticeship Council will arrange a transfer for you to another salon. You cannot be forced to go to somebody you don't like, and in any case such a transfer is only necessary in exceptional circumstances.

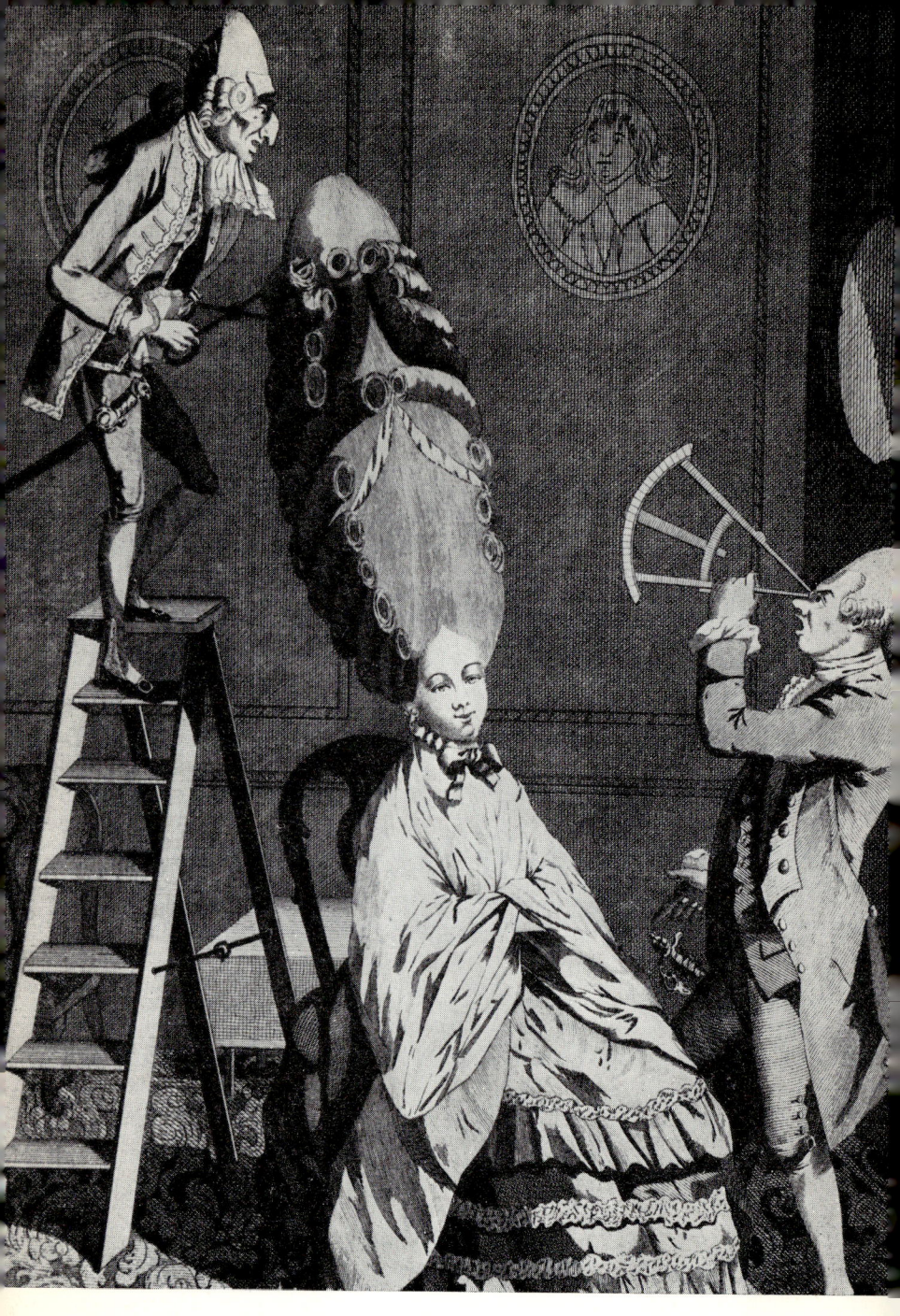

It is easier nowadays!

Apprentices watch and ask questions for the first few months, and then they start learning to do one another's hair. Good salons spend one night a week teaching their apprentices. Apart from cutting, shampooing, tinting and styling, you will have to learn how to look after and order the stores, how to keep an appointments book accurately and tidily, how to do simple book-keeping, how to make out accurate bills and how to measure clients for wigs and switches (this last is called 'boardwork').

Here is the Practical Salon Training which the National Apprenticeship Council says employers must give their apprentices:

GENTLEMEN'S HAIRDRESSING

First Year: The employer shall describe to the apprentice the care and correct use of gowns, brushes, combs and scissors. Shaving, razor setting and stropping. Plain haircutting, club and taper cutting. Dressing the hair; shampoos (wet and dry).

Second Year: Haircutting to style; trimming long hair and tapering with scissors. Moustache and beard trimming (simple style); shaving with use of steam towel: shampoos (oil, etc.); vibro massage. High frequency; hand massage for face and scalp.

Third Year: Advanced practice in styling; all razor, electric clipper and scissor haircutting. Moustache and beard trimming; shaving with the use of sponge followed by vibro treatment. Advanced face and scalp massage. The use and application of friction. The manner of operating the blow wave technique. The trimming of children's hair (any style).

LADIES' HAIRDRESSING

First Year: The employer shall describe to the apprentice the care and correct use of all instruments, brushes, combs, scissors, and all electrical equipment. The correct method of brushing and combing. The cutting and tapering of hair. Explanation of the various types of shampoo and in what manner they cleanse the hair. The employer shall explain the application of colour rinses; elementary iron curling and waving.

Second Year: Elementary permanent waving and water

waving; elementary dyeing, tinting and bleaching. Continued training in iron waving; haircutting and tapering.
Third Year: Advanced practice and training in permanent waving; hair-colouring, decolouring and bleaching. Cutting hair to style; head massage; cutting and styling children's hair.

While you are training, your employer has to let you off for one day a week, or two half-days, for training at a technical college or some other similar place. If there are not any daytime classes in your district your employer has to let you go home early on two days a week, so that you can attend evening classes. He is not allowed to take off any of your pay for the time you spend at these classes, or in going to them.

On your 'day release' you will be taught the theory of hairdressing, hygiene, some biology and chemistry, English, art, and simple book-keeping. At the end of your apprenticeship you have to take two examinations in these subjects, and your employer has to state on your Indenture that you have satisfactorily completed your three years' training. When the exam results are out and the Indenture comes back to you, you can frame it or do whatever you like with it—you are now a HAIRDRESSER!

2. *Training at a Technical College* takes two years. Here you will be given instruction and practice in cutting and treating hair, and some general educational subjects, but you will not, of course, learn anything much about the running of a salon or how to deal with clients. This is a good way to train if you feel you would be too shy to go straight to a salon, and to ask questions and find things out for yourself.

Whether or not you can easily get a job after a Technical College training depends, of course, upon the district you want to work in, but in certain areas hairdressers do not like taking junior assistants who have only been trained at a Technical College. It is important to inquire about this at several salons before deciding which is the better way for you to train.

You will not, of course, be paid if you go to a Technical College, but the tuition is free for those living in the district, and you might be able to get a grant towards your keep, depending upon your parents' income. This, too, is something to inquire about from your Local Education Department. You can find out the address from the Town Hall.

There are also a number of private training schools which say they can teach you to be a hairdresser in six months. They charge high fees, but they are not recognized by the National Hairdressers' Federation, and usually the training they give you is neither good nor complete. It stands to reason that you cannot learn all the many sides of hairdressing in a few months, and you would still have to go as an apprentice after that. So if you are really keen to become a good hairdresser, you would be wise to take up an apprenticeship at a good salon, and at the same time to continue your general education on one day a week at a Technical College. You can join the College clubs and societies, even though you are not a full-time student.

Hairdressers do not only work in salons. If you are well-trained, speak pleasantly and look nice you might find an interesting hairdressing job in a liner, a television or film studio, a theatre, a hospital or a wigmaker's.

A hairdresser working at home in 1690

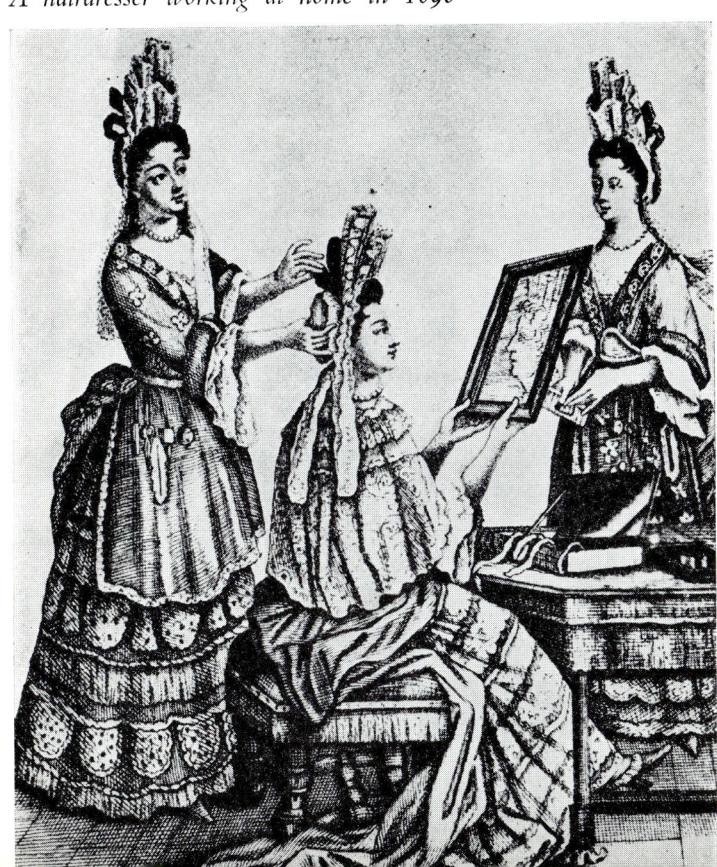

CHAPTER TEN

Your own hair

Hair is the most important part of anyone's appearance—a man's as much as a woman's. Nowadays more people than ever before bother about their looks and can afford to spend time and money in making themselves look nice.

Fashion is a strange thing. If you look back at the pictures in the earlier chapters you will probably find it difficult to realize that every single style was smart and attractive in its time. There seems to be no limit to what human beings can do to alter their appearance and it seems that everything has been tried at one time or another.

The main thing about fashion is that it *changes*. We all get tired of our hair styles and our clothes and we all need a change now and then to pep us up. Most of us don't want to look just like everybody else, but we don't want to look totally *unlike* everybody else either. We may like a new style and enjoy fitting our face and our figure to it, but when the style becomes very popular we may begin to feel that it is 'ordinary', and then we want to have something new, something different. We are never satisfied for long, and perhaps this is a good thing.

But if we are sensible there are limits to being 'in fashion'. In your hairstyle, as in the clothes you wear, it is no good being smart and with-it if what you choose does not suit you. You can camouflage your looks to a certain extent, but you cannot alter them completely: you cannot change the size or shape of your face or your head, the length of your neck, the texture of your skin and hair, and so on. If you are short you will certainly look taller with a high hairdo, but if you have a narrow thin face the high hairdo won't suit you. We all have to learn what we can and what we can't do to improve our looks; when you look at the pictures in a fashion magazine and see somebody with their hair done in a new way it is a good idea to decide for yourself: 'yes, I could do my hair that way perhaps' or 'no, that isn't for me'.

To choose a style which makes you look your best isn't easy, but it is something that comes as you get older—or which ought to, anyway. The most important thing is to *know yourself*. This means looking at yourself critically, until you know which are your good points and which are your bad ones. It means *thinking* when you go to have your hair cut, and when you buy clothes, and not being fooled by an assistant or by anybody else who says stupid, untrue things to try to get you to spend money. It also means being adventurous and willing to make mistakes sometimes. We all make mistakes and often they can be our best teachers. A new style of haircut or a new hair colour which turn out badly are not final. Hair grows again surprisingly quickly and even a 'permanent' hair colour very soon disappears. And now that wigs and 'pieces' are so much cheaper than they used to be camouflage is very easy.

To know yourself means, first of all, having a good mirror in a good light. It need not be a large mirror, though that is nice; it need not be in a room of your own, though that is nice too; but it must be somewhere where you can really *see*. Sometimes, when I look up at bedroom windows from the street and see them almost covered with curtains and with a huge dressing-table in front of them, I wonder to myself, 'how on earth does anybody know what they really look like if they dress in that room?' Do make sure that you really *can* see yourself.

You need to observe too, and that is more complicated. Have you a square chin? a sulky mouth? a low forehead? small eyes? a long nose? large ears? a short neck? spiky hair? (I don't, of course, mean all these *together*, or you really would have a problem with yourself!) Most people have both bad points and good ones, and it is sensible to be sure which are which.

For example, if your face is square or round you need to be careful not to make it look broader. In that case you need a little extra height and it will be a good idea to arrange your hair so that it curls either inwards towards your cheeks, or upwards towards your forehead. And, of course, you must not wear high necklines.

On the other hand, if your face is long and thin, width at the sides will help to widen it and probably a full fringe will suit you.

Of course there are dozens of other shapes of face and kinds of hair. Look at these sketches and see if you can decide whether or not the hairstyles suit the faces.

The best help of all in deciding how to do your hair is a frank friend—somebody who is friendly and helpful but who tells the truth even if it is not complimentary. You are very lucky indeed if you have somebody like that: others always see us more clearly than we can see ourselves. This is because when we look in a mirror we always pose a little, even if we don't mean to; other people see us when we are moving, when we are sad or happy, tired or angry, and that is the real you and the real me.

Whatever hairstyle you decide on, your hair will never look nice unless you brush it regularly and it is clean and healthy. Dull, dry, brittle hair means that you are tired or ill, or that your hair is not washed often enough. Your scalp, like the rest of your skin, produces oil all the time and when you brush and comb your hair this oil spreads down it, making it glossy and smooth.

In your teens your glands sometimes produce too much oil and then your hair gets lank and greasy and your scalp gets choked up with oil and dust. This often causes pimples on your forehead and at your hair-line and if you are not careful these may spread. A good hair wash and a thorough rinse will get rid of the extra oil, and you should do this once a week at least. As you get older you will probably find that your hair is drier and does not need to be washed so often.

You must use a good shampoo or what is called 'soft' soap. Never use household detergents or washing powders for your shampooing, because they are much too strong and would irritate your scalp and damage your hair. Too frequent shampooing is bad too and makes hair lifeless and brittle.

Don't dry your hair in front of a very hot fire if you can help it, because this may make it frizzy and dull-looking. Best of all, if you can manage it, is to dry your hair outside in the fresh air and sunshine. The chief enemy to your hair is, of course, scurf or dandruff. This looks horrid, spoils your clothes and is a sign of unhealthy hair. It is very infectious, too, and so you should not borrow or lend brushes or combs, rollers or clips, and make sure your own are washed frequently.

Nowadays, just as in the seventeenth century, there are a lot of grown-ups who complain about the length of young people's hair—and especially boys' hair. Probably it is not really the length they mind, but the untidy, unkempt, dirty hair that some boys and even girls seem to think is nice. Do remember that you can look attractive with long hair or short hair, straight hair or curly hair, but you can *never never* look attractive with dirty hair. A young, smiling, friendly face is always attractive—especially when it is framed by healthy, well kept hair.

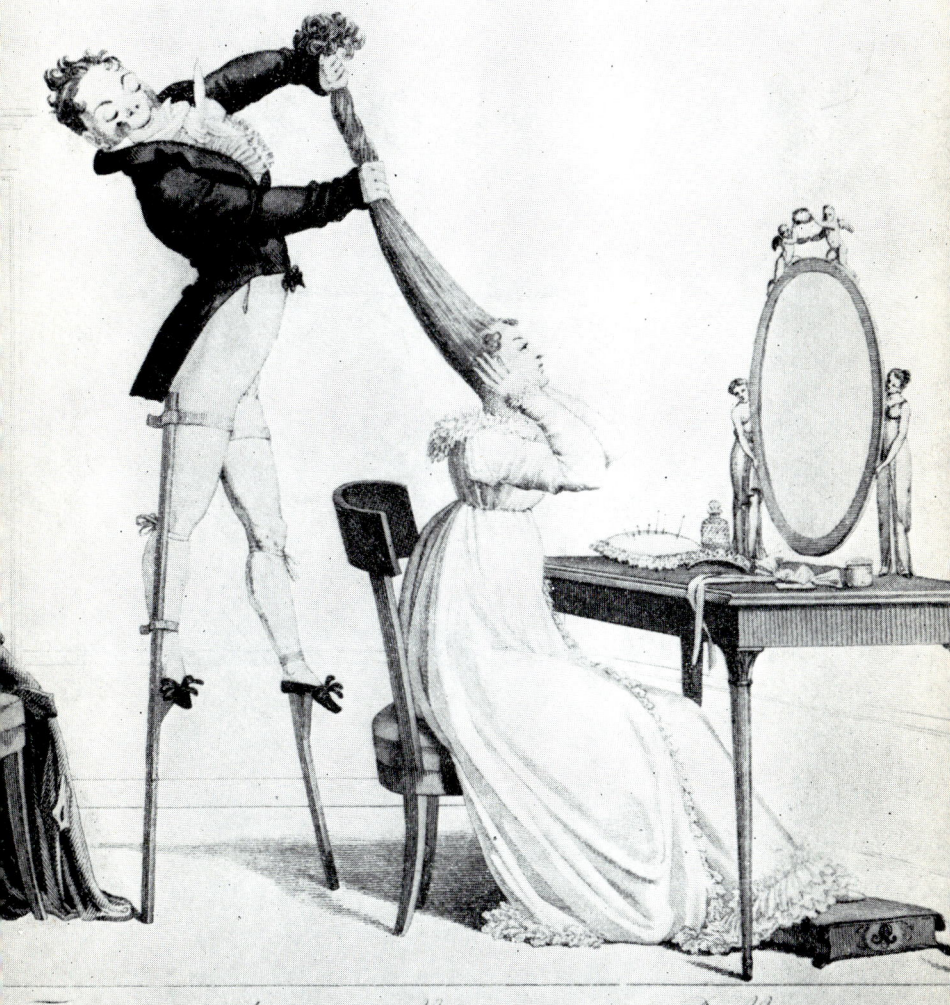

Faut apprendre à souffrir pour être Belle.

Finding out for yourself

In Chapter 8 we discussed how we can know about the dress and hairstyles that people used to wear. How much evidence can *you* find? Many places which seem dull or difficult at first, become interesting when you have a *purpose*, that is when you are looking for something special. The following is a list of places where you will be able to find evidence of how people have dressed and done their hair over the years.

Art galleries	Paintings show us both hairstyles and costumes. The postcards and booklets which are always on sale in galleries could form the basis of an interesting collection.
Museums	Many museums show costumes and some of them put the clothes onto figures which show hairstyles too.
Churches	If you explore, you will find in most churches examples of the hairstyles and costumes of different periods. These may be as statues, as carvings in wood, metal or stone or in stained-glass windows.
Plays	When you go to the theatre or cinema, or watch plays on the television, look out for details of costume and hairstyles in plays set in the past. Producers are very careful to be accurate in these details.
Books	There are not many books dealing with hair, but books on costume have many ideas to give us. Among those with the most interesting pictures are: *Picture Books of English Costume* published by the Gallery of English Costume, Manchester *Picture Books* published by the Geffrye Museum, London

A Picture History of Costume by P. Cunnington published by Studio Vista
English Costume by D. Yarwood published by Batsford.

You can find out where there are interesting places to visit when looking for historical costumes and hairstyles from the following booklets:
Historic Houses, Castles and Gardens in Great Britain and Ireland published yearly by Index Publications
Museums and Art Galleries in Great Britain and Ireland published yearly by Index Publications
Country Houses Open to the Public published by Country Life
National Trust Properties published by the National Trust.

Index

Alice bands 40
Alice in Wonderland 40
America 9
Apollo's knots 38
apprenticeship 55–60
antimacassar 36
artificial flowers 37

balls 29
bangs 40
barrister 26
beard 14, 35, 46
Beau Brummell 34
Bedford, Duke of 12–13, 50
bob 44, 45
boy's hairstyles 9–15, 22–27, 34–36, 47
braids 42
Brutus crop 26, 32
bun 38, 41

cabbage head 18, 19
careers in hairdressing 53–61
care of hair 64
caul 39
Cavaliers 11
Charles I 10, 11, 17
Charles II 12, 50
chignon 38, 39, 41, 42
Cristy cut 45
cinema, influence of 46
Civil War 10
clergymen 23, 26
combs 14, 18, 21
coronation curls 45
Crimean War 35
Cromwell, Oliver 18

dandies 34
decorations for hair 11, 17, 18, 19–20, 29, 30, 31, 37, 38–39, 40, 44
deodorants 47
Dickens, Charles 36
doctors 26
documentation 48–52
dress fashions 10, 17, 34, 41, 42, 45
dressing gown 14
dress shield 47
Dundreary whiskers 35

earrings 11, 37
eighteenth century hairstyles 22–27, 28–33
Elizabeth I 9
Eton crop 45
examinations 60

fashion dolls 33
fashion magazines 30, 33, 62
ferronière 38
First World War 43, 44
fontanges 19, 41
  fontange cap 19–20
Fontanges, Duchesse de 19
France 12, 21, 25, 32, 37
French Revolution 25, 32, 34, 37, 44

girl's hairstyles 17–21, 28–33, 37–43

hair colouring 25, 29, 39, 40, 41, 42, 46
hairdressers 14, 21, 43, 45, 48, 52, 53–61

69

hairdressing equipment   14, 21, 38,
   39, 40, 41, 48, 59
hair tidy   42
Harlow, Jean   46
Harvard College   9
hats   12, 15, 18
headache band   44
head   17
hedgehog   26, 32
hurluberlu   18, 19
hygiene   14–15, 20, 29, 33, 34, 35,
   45, 47, 64

jerseys   42
judges   26

kiss curl   17

Langtry, Lily   41
Lenglen, Suzanne   44
Little Lord Fauntleroy   36
Lister, Lord   20
Loelia, Duchess of Westminster   42
Louis XIV   19, 28
lovelock   11, 17
macaronis   24, 34
make-up   20, 33, 37–38, 40, 43,
   46–47
Marcel waving   41
Marlborough, Duke of   23
Maria-Antoinette   32
mask   33
master hairdresser   56
men's hairstyles   9–15, 22–27, 34–
   36, 46, 47
middle ages   45, 50
military hairstyles   22, 23, 26, 35
Ministry of Labour   56
moustache   35, 46
   cavalry moustache   35
museum   48, 49, 52

National Apprenticeship Council
   57, 59

National Hairdressers' Federation
   61
Nessler, Karl   42
net   39, 40
Nightingale, Florence   35
nineteenth century hairstyles   34–
   36, 37–43

page boy   45
Pasteur, Louis   20
patches   20
   patch boxes   33
Pepys, Samuel   14
perfume   14, 20, 29, 33, 35–36
permanent waving, Nestlé   42
   machineless   45
   for men   46
photography   49
Piccadilly weapers   35
picture evidence   49, 50
pole screen   27
political parties   11, 20, 25–26
pomade   13
Pompadour, Madame de   28
   style   28
porcelain   25
powder   9, 11, 13, 14, 25, 26, 29
powdering room   14
Pre-Raphaelite influence   40
private training schools   61
puff   30, 42
Puritans   11, 18

queue   23, 26

Regent, Prince   34
ribbon of convenience   19
rollers   14
rouge and pearl   38
Roundheads   11
Rousseau, Jean-Jacques   25, 32
royal coachmen   26
Royalists   11, 18
Royal Welsh Fusiliers   26

scratcher 30
Second World War 44, 46
sedan chairs 20
Selfridges 43
seventeenth century hairstyles 9-15, 17-21
shampoo 45, 64
sheep style 17
Sheridan 32
shingle 45
snood 47
suntan 47

tax 26
technical college training 60-61
teddy boy 46
tobacco 14-15
topknot 42
training grant 60-61
tulle 30
twentieth century hairstyles 45-47

Verney, Sir Ralph 21
victim's hair 33
Victoria, Queen 40, 41

waterfall 40
Wedgwood 25
wigs 12-15, 22, 23, 25-27, 29, 30, 35, 46
 bag wig 22
 bob wig 23, 26
 Cadogan wig 23
 Ramillies wig 23
 tie wig 22
 wig stand 27
women's hairstyles 17-21, 28-33, 37-43
written evidence 50-51

young people 9, 24, 32, 36, 46, 65
youth employment office 56

71